Imagine – Learn – Exercise

I0426079

Table of Contents

Special Thanks

To my wonderful wife who enjoys exercising with me.

Preface

The purpose of this book is to introduce the reader to an alternate understanding of reality concerning exercise and nutrition. It is not simply a rehash of the old maxims 'use it or lose it' and 'eat plenty of fruits and vegetables.' Many readers will learn concepts here for the first time about the magic of the universe and how to bring that wonderful energy into their lives to be transformed towards their full potential, and thus to be sources of positive energy to their immediate environment. Additionally, they will be able to do things around the house with less chance of injury, greater ease, and the satisfaction of spending their money how they see fit rather than giving it all to the healthcare system and the pharmaceutical conglomerates.

I am not including a long list of illustrations. Use your imagination. As you begin exercising and stretching you will naturally be inclined to experiment. You will discover maneuvers which tag the muscle or nerve that's got you hurting. I believe this to be the best. To be sure, variety is the key to bodybuilding progress. Thus it may be advantageous to investigate. Learn some of the various techniques espoused by the many practitioners of balanced body-building.

A few notes on sources:

1. I found a lot of my nutrition and supplement information at www.webmd.com and www.wikipedia.org

2. I have been accumulating this knowledge over the course of decades – hence some of it is common sense to dedicated workout enthusiasts, and most of it is covered in health tip sections every month in every magazine.

3. I encourage the reader to investigate further by searching the internet for proof. In the process of searching for information, one learns five times as much as he/she had originally intended.

4. If the reader does not have access to the internet or a library, then a long list of references will make little difference. Just accept that what is written is true enough to aid you in your quest for health, harmony, and balance.

Introduction

My name is Vincent DeGruy. I don't have the finest body in the land, but I am in pretty good shape. I am 38 at the time of publishing this book. My resting heart rate is about 50bpm. My blood pressure is around 115/85. I can bench press 275 for 5 reps, deadlift 345 for 5 reps, and do 5 perfect form wide grip pull-ups holding a 25 pound weight between my knees. Those weights won't get me any scholarships, awards, or trophies; unless I can still do them when I become a senior citizen (which is precisely my plan). I am probably ADD. I get bored easily. Boring work makes me sleepy. Social chit chat generally bores me. I get sleepy and close my eyes and dream about fantastic adventures. I used to try to keep my eyes open during social events. However, after learning of Lyndon B. Johnson's habit of sleeping while people were talking, I discontinued the struggle to stay awake. I've noticed also that many of us attempt to fight the sluggish sleepy feeling by snacking on high sugar foods. If possible, just close your eyes and rest. The next best thing is a piece of fruit; not a whole fruit. Fruit has sugar, but it is natural and it will make you healthy. Fruit also has vitamins and fiber. I also learned that Da Vinci took naps. I also learned that the subconscious mind processes a lot of data in different ways during sleep. This in turn helps the waking mind solve problems and gain fresh insight into the nature of things. My mind thinks about everything all the time. I change my mind a lot, and I have a lot of 'great' ideas. A little research usually reveals many shortcomings in those great ideas. God bless the internet. I weigh about 184 pounds and I am 5' 8". The only trophy I ever won was for Bible knowledge at Discovery Youth Camp in Texas. I never lasted long in sports. I hated to be coached. I didn't want to get a physical. I didn't like running. I especially didn't want to run in the summer, which I considered free time. Thankfully, my folks made my brother Jason and I go outdoors a lot. I am sure that the long periods spent outdoors contributed to a healthy immune system. Fortunately, we never ended up dead from the dumb things we did as kids. We swam in the Trinity River where it passed under Highway 360 in Arlington, TX. That was about two miles from where we lived in South Euless. Most of that area was unincorporated at the time. We rode our bicycles all over town and out to the motorcycle trails near the river. We had our fair share of scrapes. We also had a trampoline, a bunch of trees to climb, some ropes hanging from the trees, and some mean dogs. The dogs forced Jason and me to walk along fence tops or run like heck if we wanted to get to the trampoline. We had a really fun time with a rope hanging down off-center over the trampoline. We would swing out in an arc and come back to the trampoline. One of the dogs would jump and try to bite us as we swung out over the grass. He never got us, but he managed to put a hole in the seat of the jeans of one of our less lucky friends. I would practice jumping off the trampoline as high as I could go with the idea that if I were running from pursuers one day, I would be well prepared for a successful getaway. Jason and I played Kung Fu and Pro Wrestling on the trampoline and we each took our fair share of getting knocked out of the ring.

What is Your Point Vincent?

So what? My point is that we participated in lot of physical activity. Most kids are naturally energetic. They want to do something, to learn something, to have fun. The physiology of humans is fine tuned for physical and mental activity. We have a nearly infinite range of movement combinations. We have a completely infinite amount of knowledge from which to learn many things. Balance is the key. We are not designed to sit down in a square box all day. Our brains are capable of great mental activity while sitting in the box, but the body must be catered to as well. For it is the body which nourishes the brain. It is physical activity which strengthens the body.

One day while sitting in Momma's car, I was perusing the 1980 Guinness Book of World Records. It named Arnold Schwarzenegger as "The most perfectly developed man in the history of the world..." I was awed. I wanted to be like him. From then on, whenever I was at the grocery store, I camped out in the magazine section until my mom or grandmother finished shopping. I would usually just read about the routines of various bodybuilders and check out their physiques. I always skipped the stuff about nutrition, considering it boring. If I ran across a magazine with Arnold in it, I had to purchase it for further study and inspiration.

I was attending Lakeview Mission Church in Fort Worth at the time. Brother Michael Bell also went to church there. His muscles were like the guys in the magazines. He was about 6' 2" 235 pounds and all muscle. He would flex his arms and let us kids hang off of them like tree limbs. He advised me to start doing push-ups and crunches every day. I figured that since I knew someone with big muscles who was giving me advice, then I could also have big muscles. So I began doing push-ups and crunches on a regular basis.

All through junior high, I didn't have much access to weights. The athletes used the weight facilities. I was shy and not familiar with the gym. When my last class ended each day, I was ready to get on my bike and hit the trails.

I signed up for gymnastics twice. On each occasion I thought it possible that being in gymnastics would somehow cause my body to be more muscular like the folks throwing themselves about the mats. I believed that I could have a physique like the gymnasts on the other end of the gym. I quit each time after about one day of witnessing the rigorous training and coaching. In tenth grade I signed up for weightlifting. I had found my ideal physical education class. I was pretty weak. My max bench press was about 120 pounds. I weighed about 135 pounds. My big goal was to bench press 135. That consists of two big 45 pound plates on a 45 pound bar ...

```
.........   --[|]----------[|]--    ........
```

```
         .........   --[|]----------[|]--    ........
```

```
                 .........   --[|]---------[|]--    .........
```

It looked cool. I kept at it. I was able to do 5 or 6 reps with 135 by the end of the school year. I hurt my neck once doing incline bench press and resolved to be more careful.

Eventually, I met Brandon Bowen as a result of going over to his house to socialize with his sister, DJ. She spoke regularly about her big brother. I disregarded it as so much fluff, thinking every girl thinks highly of her big brother. Then I met him and saw his athletic records posted at the gym. This guy was amazing. He was benching over 300 in 11th grade. He jumped higher and ran faster than most other athletes. His records were on the wall to prove it. This sort of strength and speed might be expected from a star player at a university. But Brandon was a 5' 9" sixteen year old. I knew I could learn something from him. He had some weights in his parent's garage. He gave me some literature on Bulgarian Olympic training techniques. I learned that

1. 45 minutes of lifting was plenty
2. 4-6 sets of 6-8 reps was plenty
3. After 45 minutes, you are probably eating into your recovery time.

He also stressed the importance of taking in more nutrition around the clock. About this time, I also read about how some bodybuilder had started eating steaks about midnight every night and began to see great results. So I began having a protein shake late every night. They never tasted great. They never mixed well. I didn't care. I just wanted my body to look more like Conan the Barbarian. I eventually started mixing in some eggs and bananas. I had seen Sylvester Stallone drink them in Rocky. I now know about Salmonella poisoning. I recommend to never eat raw eggs. I got sick a couple times. It is very unpleasant. Consuming raw eggs is an unnecessarily risky behavior. Boil them first. They will taste better. The protein shakes today mix easily, taste great, and have plenty of nutrition. Additionally, they are inexpensive. Walmart carries a good one for about $16 which is about 30 shakes.

I continued to make small gains. When I was almost 18, I finally joined the 200 Club. That means I lifted over 200 pounds on something. For me, it was a bench press of 205 a couple of weeks before I turned 18. I still only weighed about 147.

After turning 18, I started working in restaurants as a waiter, a busboy, a cook, an assistant bartender, etc. I was also taking various classes at the community college. I thought restaurants were great for meeting girls and getting free food. I had no idea what I planned on doing with my life. I continued to work out and periodically kept a workout journal to track my progress. The way the journal was used specifically was that it allowed me to know exactly how much weight or how many reps I needed to add to the workout to demonstrate forward progress.

Part One –

Forward Progress

A fundamental truth about exercise is that you cannot possibly do everything. Don't try. Do a little every day. Observe how children play with exercise equipment. Do likewise.

That being the case, one can claim progress in a thousand ways depending on the goals and circumstances.

For example

- More reps with a certain weight
- More reps on the second or third set with a certain weight
- More weight with same number of reps
- More weight with any number of reps
- More weight with better stability
- More extra stretching between sets
- More flexing between sets

And so the list goes on. Some oft-quoted fellow said "Happiness is having goals and making progress towards them." Thus one can have an infinite number of variations and an infinite amount of progress when one begins exercising daily.

Sometimes the only progress I can claim is that I am blessed with the breath of life first, so that I may even think on it. And usually I can believe that I am about as good at any task today as I was yesterday. Thus it follows that I have indeed made progress towards the goal of doing what I can to maintain a healthy balance in my body.

Sure... I like to eat some junk food occasionally. But I must still eat some healthy stuff for my digestive systems so that they will process the junk food appropriately and efficiently.

I digress...

I reached 23 with no degree, lots of fun memories, and muscles which were still not getting huge. I never weighed over 155 pounds. I had hurt my shoulder doing heavy bench press, and hurt my neck with heavy dumbbell shoulder press and incline shrugs (lay face down on incline, arms hang down with dumbbells in hand—probably a bad idea). My elbow would hurt so badly after racquetball that the arm was useless for shifting gears in my truck. I hated getting hurt. I learned some valuable lessons.

1. Warm-up with light weights. Do some light weights for several major muscle groups. Do 15 reps with a light weight which could be lifted 20-25 times. Do them in perfect form. Feel the stretching and flexing of the muscles. Imagine the blood flowing into those groups. The body is composed of systems and teams. No muscle works alone.
   a. Pull downs – warms up the back muscles, rear shoulder muscles, biceps, and forearms
   b. Bench Press – Chest, side and front shoulders, triceps.
   c. Squats with body weight – hamstrings, glutes, quadriceps.
   d. Sit-ups or leg lifts – Abdominals play a key role in everything as well.
2. Add a few pounds at a time for the first few sets to get the muscles acclimated and the blood flowing. This will also help you discover any weakness or lingering pain.
3. Spend quality time on shoulder exercises. Use the cables to exercise your rotator cuff every month. You will never regret it.

4. Alternate between heavy and light workouts. Do heavy for 2 or 3 workouts, then go light for 2 or 3 workouts.
5. Heavy workouts put a lot of stress on tendons, ligaments, and connective tissues. They will get injured if you do not give them a break.
6. Light workouts improve the body's ability to get oxygen and other nutrients into the muscles.
7. Alternate hands on racquetball. This is hard at first, but it is great for the brain and for creating balance and reducing the stress concentration in the dominant arm.
8. Stretching should be done after the light weights. Intense stretching before lifting is less effective and more likely to cause injury. Stretching after warm ups and during lifting will cause muscles to become more flexible and will increase the size of the muscle for the blood to flow into it and make it bigger.

I define a heavy workout as one where you plan to workout with your 5 rep max. A light workout is when you lift a weight that you can lift at least 15 reps.

Then my luck with results changed. I came across a copy of Sports Supplement Review by Bill Phillips. It changed my life. I had discovered the secrets to bodybuilding success.

I designed a workout around the idea from the book that 2 weeks of a low calorie diet followed by 2 weeks on a high calorie diet will cause your testosterone, growth hormone, and Insulin-Growth-Factor-1 levels to double. Additionally, during the low calorie cycle the fat-burning phase of your metabolism will be extra effective. Both of these effects taper off back to normal after about 2 weeks.

For 5 months I would gain 15 pounds for 2 weeks, then lose 10 pounds for 2 weeks. It was like a game to me and Christopher (my coworker at the time who was also interested in building some muscle). I would exercise with progressively heavier and more intense workouts for the 2 weeks of heavy eating. Then I would keep it light with a lot of reps for the 2 weeks of low calorie diet.

I highly recommend that anybody wishing for some drastic progress try this.

Now with some fundamental assumptions cleared I boldly claim that 'We are all bodybuilders.' As long as you live, your body is creating new cells. As long as you live, your body is reacting to the stimuli placed on it by you. Muscles get stronger because they need more strength to cope with the demands which you place on them. Muscle fibers work together better as a team so that they can get work done with more efficiency and success. If you neglect to exercise, then your body will become weaker over time. Your bones become denser (hence more strong) as a reaction to you lifting weights. Your heart learns to pump blood more strongly throughout your body in response to an increased necessity to get fresh blood into an area to remove lactic acid (and other waste products) and to deliver oxygen. All of these processes are stimulated by physical activity, not sitting on a couch or laying down. To paraphrase Jack Lalanne, 'Any dumb mule can die. You must work to stay alive.'

Let us put the idea of exercise as 'work' into perspective. Our body is at work all day long. It works to turn food into energy and into the necessary building blocks of our many component systems. Exercise is living. Exercise causes your body to release endorphins which are the chemicals that give you a feel-good feeling. A person can continue to do any activity they like throughout the day. A little exercise on a regular basis creates a body that can enjoy every activity a little more; and it makes every activity easier. Exercise causes your body to release chemicals which neutralize pain and reduce inflammation. Lack of exercise allows weakness, pain, and inflammation to consume your body. These are facts. One simply has to do an internet search to discover hundreds of scientific studies proving these points.

Force Fields, Golden Particles of Energy, Vibrations, and Visualization

Visualization is not much different than imagining. When one chooses to imagine that a certain event is transpiring, it is the same as visualizing. The act of imagining creates a pattern for a possibility for a course of action for the body. Additionally, we are creators of our future. Visualizing that future causes us to make progress towards it. Read The Source Field Investigations by David Wilcock for plenty of scientific studies proving that a person's intentions make things happen in the physical universe. There are several visualizations which I use on a regular basis to move mountains in the gym. These techniques work in other areas of life as well. The gym is simply a place to practice the technique and see concrete results.

One great example which has worked very well for me goes as follows:

a) Do the light warm-ups and stretches
b) Do a couple more lifts on the exercise which is the focus of that day's work out (For example, even though my plan is to do heavy bench press, I still warm up the whole body. This will be easier to do after you have injured a shoulder, or pulled a hamstring muscle, strained a neck, etc. doing bench press; but you don't have to wait till that happens.) If I plan to lift 315 for 5 reps then I get there by the following route:

  i.   15 reps pull down 115 pounds
  ii.   15 reps bench 135 pounds
  iii. 15 reps hyperextensions (aka supermans)
  iv.   12-15 leg lifts or crunches
  v.   10-15 squats
  vi.   3 reps (very slow) bench press 225 pounds
  vii. 20 shoulder circles with 5 pounds

viii. 2 reps (perfect form) bench press 295 pounds

ix. BAM BAM BAM – Take a minute to say a prayer "Thank you Jesus for a great life, a great wife, and another opportunity to lift weights and do what I want."

x. Close right nostril and breathe through left while imagining golden particles of energy coming from any light source in the universe (including Heaven, the sun, the lights in the room, or even from the people in the gym whose attention may have wondered my way), going up through my left nostril, saturating my right side brain, going down my spine, and saturating the muscles and helper muscles involved in the upcoming heavy lift. I do the same with each nostril until I have firmly visualized it without fail.

xi. I also imagine ace bandage-like energy wraps around my shoulders and neck.

xii. I imagine a hulking energy Arnold stepping into my space.

xiii.   I imagine myself lifting the 315 pounds without fail.

xiv.   I stroll confidently back to the bench.

xv.   I lay down, close my eyes, and softly hum in such a way that I feel the noise completely engulf my brain. I am creating a force field around me with the vibrations which will affect the rotational spin of the atoms in the weights. This in turn will alter the effect of gravity on the weights. It is a small localized effect, yet enough to move what I need to move. This is how monks move huge boulders through the air in the Himalayas and how pyramids can be built. (Investigating the Source Field by David Wilcock)

xvi.   As I lay there, I once more imagine the weight going up and down as if gravity did not exist and the bar merely glided up or down energy lines at will. I might even move my hands up and down in the fashion of lifting the weight, but without the bar in my hands. Or I might just rest them near my body or on the bar feeling the power increase.

xvii. Then I do it. I have failed less than once
in a thousand times to succeed in
lifting the heavy weight. Occasionally, I
could not get all five reps by myself.
But I got a lot of work done, and I felt
like a superman.

This works for any other lift as well. Just substitute
the different lift into the place of bench press. You
can also visualize different people or a future version
of yourself. I started by visualizing Mark Wahlberg
(AKA Marky Mark) when I weighed 155 pounds.
When I was 185 -190 I moved up to bigger guys,
including a 6' 4" 285 pound Jesus of Nazareth. It is
your visualization. Use what inspires you.

These concrete results and successes in turn increase
one's strength and one's faith. It naturally follows
then that one increases in amazement at the
wonders of the universe. Each of us is capable of
wondrous achievements. Simply perusing the history
books and reading about the lifestyles and
achievements of the giants of history will enlighten
any reader. For in these books one discovers that the
people we read about encountered the same
desperate situations and challenges which we face
today.

Transformation and the Necessity of Training

The cells in our bodies are constantly transforming, and new ones are constantly created. It is therefore necessary that we train these new cells to function in a way which maximizes our potential. Every person has many desires. These include loving and being loved, being free from pain, getting things done around the house, etc. It is obvious then that having good health will make it easier for the body to have success at any one of these things. Even if a person simply wants to sit on the couch, eat chips, and watch TV, then he/she can spend more years doing these activities with good health. With regular exercise the digestive system will work more efficiently, and the metabolism will be increased. Thanks to these two effects a person can eat more of the junk desired and spend more years doing it without the negative effects on health generally associated with eating junk and being slothful.

Cancer and Heart Disease

Cancer and heart disease are the number one killers of Americans. Most Americans are scared to death of unlikely deaths and think nothing of changing their lifestyles to prevent the likely deaths. For example, many are afraid of dying in a car accident. Most police officers will tell you "I never unbuckled a corpse from a seatbelt." The lesson here is if you are wearing your seatbelt, then your chances of dying in a car wreck are very slim. If you don't exercise, your chances of dying from heart disease or cancer are very great.

Other complications of living an unhealthy life are obvious from the dramatic increase in diabetic adults and other obesity related symptoms.

Even a thin person with no weight problems should be concerned about the health of his/her bones, muscles, and organs. When a person exercises, the body becomes more optimized towards health and wellness. It gets rid of poisons. The immune system is strengthened. The heart gets stronger.

The Bare Minimum

Time spent exercising is never time wasted.

This section discusses the bare minimum of nutrition which all people should know so that they can make informed decisions, and the bare minimum of exercise which all people should do in order to keep their bodies working properly, and resistant to atrophy.

Nutrition

Drink water. It makes up 70% of the body. Water carries nutrition to cells and removes waste products. Symptoms of dehydration include:

- Dark urine
- Fatigue
- Lightheadedness
- Increased heart rate
- Overheat
- Muscle cramp
- Constipation
- Skin less elastic
- No more tears
- Thirsty

People often eat, thinking that the food will replace the unhappy feeling in their stomach with contentment. Water works better. Stop drinking sodas. Drink more water. It is your friend in the endeavor to maintain a healthy body which is resistant to disease and imbalance.

It is not about looks. It is about putting your body through the paces every day. You are the master. Your body is yours to command. Ensure that each of your parts is working properly and pain-free every day. Exercise.

The body cycles between anabolic and catabolic states. Anabolic means that protein synthesis (food turns into muscle tissue) is occurring. Catabolic means that protein breakdown (body is breaking down the proteins to use for energy or some other purpose) is occurring. Approximately 6 hours after consuming protein the body enters into a catabolic state, and the metabolism slows down. This back and forth cycle is known as Homeostasis, or 'same state.' The purpose is to maintain balance and not make inordinate amounts of progress in one direction or the other. The theory about the reason for this cycling back and forth is that if a person's body was always in an anabolic state, he would soon be so muscular that he could not possibly eat enough to maintain his mass. Theories aside, the fact remains.

- The body cycles back and forth between anabolic and catabolic states. The catabolic state begins approximately 6 hours after consuming protein.

This is important to know. First of all, it is a bad idea to attempt to lose fat by going all day without eating. After about 6 hours the body will begin breaking down protein from the muscles to feed itself. The metabolism slows down. Fat burning slows down. The body believes that a time of famine has arrived. Consequently, the fat is saved for later and the muscles are consumed.

The point is this:

- Consume some protein every 6 hours at the minimum. It will keep your metabolism working at a high rate, and it will preserve muscle mass.
- Muscles use more calories per hour than fat tissue. The increased calorie burning and muscle mass will work together to make your fat disappear, or at least not get worse.

Exercise

Every morning I do a simple warm-up to keep all my muscles healthy and up to the minimum standards of healthy living. It is as follows:

- 50 Push-ups
- 40 leg lifts (laying on back, lift feet up and down between 3 and 15 inches)
- 20 Scissor lifts (laying on back, put feet straight up in the air, lift butt an inch or two pushing the legs straight up a little; and reach out with fingers towards toes.)

- 20 bicycles (laying on back -feet moving in motion of bicycle; elbows and shoulders moving off of ground to meet knees in alternating fashion)
- 15-20 Squats (knees going in circles to maintain flexibility) Also doing some wide leg sumo-style squats to stretch groin area.
- Bent over one-arm dumbbell rows (two feet on ground, one hand on a support structure)
- 10 outstretched hand circles (for shoulders)
- 3 Full range of motion head circles
- 20 Dumbbell shrugs
- 30 Dumbbell shoulder press
- 15 Dumbbell biceps supinating curls
- 15 Dumbbell overhead tricep extensions

This is a short easy workout. I do it with 25 pound dumbbells. Someone who is just starting to be an everyday workout artist would use less weight and less reps. For example, one might start with 10 pushups, 10 leg raises and 10 squats. Every week add a few repetitions. After a couple of months start doing some light dumbbell work. One could also use some resistance bands (stretchy bungee-like cord).

Let me be clear. When I wake up, I do not feel like exercising. I want to go back to sleep or just lay there.

The **TRUTH** about feelings is this –

'*Feelings come and go. I still have things to do.*'

I set my alarm for 40 minutes before I have to leave for work.

- I get up,
- go into the kitchen,
- turn on the lights (bright lights stimulate the brain into waking up)
- turn on the coffee,
- add water to protein mix (fast and easy)
- shake and drink protein shake (to immediately take my body out of a catabolic state)
- put food into small cooler for my day's sustenance,
- make cup of coffee (caffeine works)
- And begin exercising.

The night before, I have laid out my clothes. I have also portioned my food for the next day. It does not have to be rocket science. Some ham and bread will work just fine. Fish, greens, and mashed potatoes will be even better.

When I am done exercising, I feel pumped up and healthy. If I don't exercise again that day, I take comfort knowing I have done the bare minimum. I have done this for about 10 years every day. Getting the blood flowing creates a sense of well-being by

a) Releasing endorphins
b) Removing toxins from the body
c) Putting fresh oxygen into the body through stimulated breathing
d) Drawing energy into the body – remember that focusing on your health creates health and attracts energy

One final thought about the bare minimum. When I consider not exercising because I am tired or sore or whatever, an ever-present question,

"Is today going to be the day that I choose to embrace declining health? Is today going to be the day when my willpower gets weak and I can't make my body do the same amount of work as it did yesterday?"

And the answer is <u>ALWAYS</u> a great big resounding **NO**! Today is not that day. If I have worked especially hard all week I may take longer to do the work, but it will get done every day. I may even cut back some on the reps occasionally, but I still do every exercise. And I usually go to the gym later in the day on the days where I did a few less reps in the morning.

This is the bare minimum. I strongly suggest that every reader begin very soon on some sort of daily bare minimum routine for your own benefit.

Pre and Post Exercise Nutrition

The minutes and hours before and after exercise are very important. First, decide the primary goals for a particular exercise session.

A. Fat loss – When the goal is fat loss, the best bet is to wait 3 or 4 hours after consuming a meal to exercise. Exercising immediately after eating (or within 2 hours) is more likely to use the nutrition which was just consumed for energy, rather than stored fat. 3-4 hours after eating one is more likely to burn accumulated fat deposits. Generally speaking, a person will be weaker at this time. I mean weaker as in able to lift less weight.

B. Muscle Building – About an hour after eating solid food [or immediately after consuming liquid food (aka protein shake) – since it digests quickly] is a good time to begin a workout for the purpose of building muscle. A person will be strongest about 1½ - 2 hours after a meal (or 30 – 45 minutes after a shake). If the goal is to build muscle and be at your strongest, then definitely consume some nutrition before the exercise session (1½- 2 hours for solid food and 30-45 minutes for liquid food).

C. General fitness/endurance – The timing of the pre-workout meal is not so important for general fitness or endurance training. Endurance is primarily a mental thing. Physiologically speaking though, endurance limits go down the further one gets from nutrition. But he/she can make great strides in maintaining cardiovascular (heart pumping blood and lungs oxygenating blood) fitness regardless of the timing of the last meal.

Part Two – Possible Workout Routines

Office Person Workout

This section is for the lucky few who have a gym at the office, but don't want to bother with the hassle of changing clothes, getting sweaty, showering, and all that jive. We all know that sitting in front of a computer all day is unhealthy, even if furnished with the best ergonomic chair and keyboard. For myself, after putting a few numbers into a spreadsheet, I am ready to go straight to sleep. Sometimes I do. I stand up, walk out to my Jeep Grand Cherokee, put down the back seat, lay down, take off my shoes, put on my headphones, listen to the soothing sound of rain and church bells, wrap a towel around my head to shut out the world, and pass out. 10 – 15 minutes later, I am re-energized. I actually use Holosync technology (look it up). They have overlaid the music with some tones which pump a different tone into each ear so that the mind enters into a state similar to deep meditation. It never fails to deliver me to a refreshed state 10 – 15 minutes after laying down. I can't work sleepy.

Enough about naps. Here is the 411 on a great exercise strategy for the office place, which avoids getting sweaty, produces amazing results, and keeps a person living well all day long. Go to the gym for about 3-5 minutes once every 90-120 minutes. I present the reader with a practical easy to follow guide for a Monday thru Friday exercise plan.

	Light Duty Weeks		**Heavy Duty Weeks**
Mon	Deadlifts (1 set x 12 reps) Shrugs (1 x 12) Elliptical Trainer (2-3 minutes)		Same as light duty with additional heavier set of deadlifts and shrugs after elliptical trainer. (First set is like a warm-up)
Tues	Bench (1 x 15) Shoulder Press (1 x 15) Elliptical Trainer (2-3 minutes)		Same as light duty with additional heavier set of Bench and Shoulder Press after elliptical trainer. (First set is like a warm-up)
Wed	Pull-ups(or Pull-downs) Abs (15-20 reps) Elliptical Trainer (2-3 minutes)		Same as light duty with additional heavier set of Pull-Ups after elliptical

			trainer. (First set is like a warm-up)
Thurs	Bicep Curls (1 x 15) Abs (15-20 reps) Elliptical Trainer (2-3 minutes)		Same as light duty with additional heavier set of curls after elliptical trainer. (First set is like a warm-up)
Fri	Tricep Press (1 x 15) Abs (15-20 reps) Elliptical Trainer (2-3 minutes)		Same as light duty with additional heavier set of tricep extension after elliptical trainer. (First set is like a warm-up)

Notes about some of the items in the schedule:

- It is a good idea to have some variety to keep the body stimulated. By having light and heavy duty weeks, a person can focus some weeks on strength training, while focusing other weeks on cardiovascular fitness.
- Each workout should only be 3-5 minutes in duration. Afterward, drink some cold water and take off your shoes to cool down.
- Use a weight which could easily be lifted for 20 reps. Except for the second set on heavy

duty weeks; then use something which requires a little work to get 10-15 reps.

- Visit the gym 4-5 times in a day, doing the same exercises each time for that day.
- Hang from the pull-up bar for a great spine decompression. Try to touch your chest with your chin and your back with the back of your head for some incredible stretch and flexibility relief. Swing your feet as if walking on air to really inject some relief into your spinal column.
- Make pull-ups easy by putting a foot against the backrest. Pull-ups are hard and can be thought of as heavy weight for 99% of the population. Good form with light weight will be very beneficial.
- Deadlifts cure back problems and weakness of the will. You are literally developing some backbone and willpower by doing deadlifts every week. Deadlifts strengthen core strength. Just do it.
- Always keep your eyes focused in front and slightly up to prevent neck strains and improve blood flow (energy flow) to the areas being exercised.

- Any substitutions are fine. The point is to focus on a different muscle each day, and do a little cardio each day. It adds up. It keeps the metabolism going.

Got No Money Workouts

Got no money? Keep it simple. You have plenty of time. Of that I am sure. Let us move on.

Staying fit is like a nonsense phrase. I prefer to think in terms of staying balanced. So I have a healthy low intensity stretch and exercise routine which is actually very good.

1. Do some push-ups.
2. Do some ab exercises
3. Do some squats and deadlifts
4. Do some yoga
5. Eat some
6. Drink some water.

If you are not able to spend any money for the gym or on fitness equipment for the house, then staying healthy should be a top priority so that you can be ready:

a) To spend the money you are making
b) To continue persevering through what trials and tribulations may come your way.

Got Less Than $20 Workouts

Less than $20 is no problem. You can move mountains with $20 worth of stuff. Next chance you get, go to Academy or some other sporting goods store. You can find some resistance bands for about $5-$7. Look around. See what wonderful things can be purchased in the market place. Check Amazon and you never have to leave home.

Resistance bands are amazing. Put them around the bed posts and get to work on all sorts of stuff which immediately comes to mind when you lay your hands and attention on to the purpose of your endeavors.

Got Enough Time/Money Workouts

Exercise at leisure. Put in some work every month on stabilizer muscles and stretch regularly. When you want to go a little harder in the gym, a little past failure, and you don't have a spotter handy, it's no big deal. Here are some tips for the solo workout artist on forced reps:

- Rest a couple of seconds – Then do some more reps
- Take off some of the weight – Then do some more reps
- Go extra slow sometimes

- Do light work for the small stabilizer muscles (like stretching the shoulders and rotator cuff while warming up for bench press).

Always experiment with new ways to challenge yourself. Seek to improve in any weak areas. Think about what you are doing. Stop counting. Stop thinking about the TV, the phone, and the car. Just exercise. Let your mind be free from plotting, planning, and postulating.

Likewise, think about the muscles involved in an exercise. Let us imagine that one morning, as I am doing push-ups, I choose to really experience the push-up and, simultaneously, choose not to concentrate on counting. The thoughts which might occur to me are thus:

- What is happening?
- What can I do with these push-ups?
  - First six inches of a full push-up for several repetitions
  - First 12 inches?
  - 12 inches for 35 reps, followed by 18 in. X 10 reps, followed by 5 reps doing just the last 9 inches of a full push-up?
- What can I do with some leg-raises? Does the position of my feet make much difference?

- o A lot. And yes.
- o As you lay on your back with your feet resting on the ground, put your hands on your mid-section.
- o Start moving one or both feet to different locations and elevations.
- o You will definitely feel with your hands how some of your different muscles in the mid-section tense up to move your foot which is 3 feet away.
- o And so you learn and do what feels best to you.

Got All Day Workouts

These are some helpful tips.

1. Drink a little water every 2-3 hours.
2. Stretch whatever ails you.
3. Do the bare minimum.
4. Experiment with the resistance cord

In reality, we all have all day. Most days. There is only one day in our life when we have less than 24 hours. We should then strive to keep our bodies ready to enjoy the miracles that may come.

Then why count?

I don't really think that counting is necessary for simple exercises for one's own health.

Perhaps it focuses the left and right brains onto some present task and carries a person from beginning of activity to end. Counting is then like a bridge.

Should I count reps..., breaths..., or other arbitrary countables?

Numbers are neutral. There is much to be said for the Scientific Method.

Count as a distraction to your present pain.

Count so that you can have a number to work towards.

Count because gravity is pushing down on everything and you want to know how much weight you can throw around, and how many times you can do it in a certain amount of time.

Or don't count.

The important thing is to make your body move. Then you can focus on what the muscle feels like. What exactly is happening there after a few reps?

Part Three – Words about Exercise

Facts/Factoids/Fantasies

1. "Sweating is losing weight" – The truth is that sweating is the body's way of releasing heat and cooling down. It is like the body's air conditioner. The water traps heat. The water comes out through the sweat gland. The heat comes out with it. The body is losing heat and water. This is not the kind of weight loss which is important. Exercise does increase metabolism and burn calories. Burn more calories than you consume and weight is lost. 3500 calories equals one pound.

2. "If I start lifting weights, I will become bulky or possibly inflexible." - Wrong. You will not accidentally become bulky. Bulking up requires a lot of dedication, a lot of protein that you probably don't normally ingest, and a lot of weightlifting. Some regular low intensity weight lifting will strengthen and tone your muscles. It will make them work properly. It will increase the density of your bones, to help you avoid osteoporosis. It will speed up your metabolism. There are no negative side effects. Only positive side

effects result from exercise. Stretching regularly will prevent inflexibility.

3. "I don't need to work out. I do work all day at my job." – Wrong again. Doing work all day at your job is a form of spending your energy. Exercising channels energy into you. It increases your body's ability to do more work and to be healthy and balanced. When you exercise you are focusing on self. You are training your cells to operate at a higher level of energy and vitality.

4. "Cardiovascular exercise is the best way to burn fat" – Wrong. Though it is about 15% true. A person can lift weights in a cardiovascular way by not resting a lot between sets. He/she can do some light stretching/flexing in between sets or some light exercises on other muscles to keep the heart rate up.

Insulin

Insulin information is straight from Wikipedia.

Insulin is a peptide hormone, produced by beta cells of the pancreas, and is central to regulating carbohydrate and fat metabolism in the body. Insulin causes cells in the liver, skeletal muscles, and fat tissue to absorb glucose (sugar) from the blood. In the liver and skeletal muscles, glucose is stored as glycogen, and in fat cells it is stored as triglycerides.

Insulin stops the use of fat as an energy source by inhibiting the release of glucagon. Glucagon, a peptide hormone secreted by the pancreas, raises blood glucose levels. Its effect is opposite that of insulin, which lowers blood glucose levels. The pancreas releases glucagon when blood sugar (glucose) levels fall too low. Glucagon causes the liver to convert stored glycogen into glucose, which is released into the bloodstream. High blood glucose levels stimulate the release of insulin. Insulin allows glucose to be taken up and used by insulin-dependent tissues. Thus, glucagon and insulin are part of a feedback system that keeps blood glucose levels at a stable level. With the exception of the metabolic disorder diabetes mellitus and metabolic syndrome, insulin is provided within the body in a constant proportion to remove excess glucose from the blood, which otherwise would be toxic. When blood glucose levels fall below a certain level, the body begins to use stored sugar as an energy source through glycogenolysis, which breaks down the glycogen stored in the liver and muscles into glucose, which can then be utilized as an energy source. As a central metabolic control mechanism, its status is also used as a control signal to other body systems (such as amino acid uptake by body cells). In addition, it has several other anabolic effects throughout the body.

When control of insulin levels fails, diabetes mellitus can result. As a consequence, insulin is used medically to treat some forms of diabetes mellitus. Patients with type 1 diabetes depend on external insulin (most commonly injected subcutaneously) for their survival because the hormone is no longer produced internally. Patients with type 2 diabetes are often insulin resistant and, because of such resistance, may suffer from a "relative" insulin deficiency. Some patients with type 2 diabetes may eventually require insulin if other medications fail to control blood glucose levels adequately. Over 40% of those with Type 2 diabetes require insulin as part of their diabetes management plan.

Synthesis, physiological effects, and degradation

Insulin is produced in the pancreas and released when any of several stimuli are detected. These stimuli include ingested protein and glucose in the blood produced from digested food. Carbohydrates can be polymers of simple sugars or they can be the simple sugars themselves. If the carbohydrates include glucose, then that glucose will be absorbed into the bloodstream and blood glucose level will begin to rise. In target cells, insulin initiates a signal transduction, which has the effect of increasing glucose uptake and storage. Finally, insulin is degraded, terminating the response.

Insulin undergoes extensive posttranslational modification along the production pathway. Production and secretion are largely independent; prepared insulin is stored awaiting secretion.

Insulin and its related proteins have been shown to be produced inside the brain, and reduced levels of these proteins are linked to Alzheimer's disease.

Release

The first phase release is rapidly triggered in response to increased blood glucose levels. The second phase is a sustained, slow release of newly formed vesicles triggered independently of sugar.

Release of insulin is strongly inhibited by the stress hormone norepinephrine (noradrenaline), which leads to increased blood glucose levels during stress.

When the glucose level comes down to the usual physiologic value, insulin release from the β-cells slows or stops. If blood glucose levels drop lower than this, especially to dangerously low levels, release of hyperglycemic hormones forces release of glucose into the blood from cellular stores, primarily liver cell stores of glycogen. By increasing blood glucose, the hyperglycemic hormones prevent or correct life-threatening hypoglycemia.

Evidence of impaired first-phase insulin release can be seen in the glucose tolerance test, demonstrated by a substantially elevated blood glucose level at 30 minutes, a marked drop by 60 minutes, and a steady climb back to baseline levels over the following hourly time points.

Oscillations

Insulin release from pancreas oscillates with a period of 3–6 minutes.

During the digestion, generally, one or two hours following a meal, insulin release from the pancreas is not continuous, but oscillates with a period of 3–6 minutes, changing from generating a blood insulin concentration more than about 800 pmol/l to less than 100 pmol/l. This is thought to avoid down-regulation of insulin receptors in target cells, and to assist the liver in extracting insulin from the blood. This oscillation is important to consider when administering insulin-stimulating medication, since it is the oscillating blood concentration of insulin release, which should, ideally, be achieved, not a constant high concentration.

Signal transduction

Special transporter proteins in cell membranes allow glucose from the blood to enter a cell. These transporters are, indirectly, under blood insulin's control in certain body cell types (e.g., muscle cells). Low levels of circulating insulin, or its absence, will prevent glucose from entering those cells (e.g., in type 1 diabetes). More commonly, however, there is a decrease in the sensitivity of cells to insulin (e.g., the reduced insulin sensitivity characteristic of type 2 diabetes), resulting in decreased glucose absorption. In either case, there is 'cell starvation' and weight loss, sometimes extreme. In a few cases, there is a defect in the release of insulin from the pancreas. Either way, the effect is the same: elevated blood glucose levels.

Activation of insulin receptors leads to internal cellular mechanisms that directly affect glucose uptake by regulating the number and operation of protein molecules (in the cell membrane) that transport glucose into the cell

Two types of tissues are most strongly influenced by insulin, as far as the stimulation of glucose uptake is concerned: muscle cells (myocytes) and fat cells (adipocytes). The former are important because of their central role in movement, breathing, circulation, etc., and the latter because they accumulate excess food energy against future needs. Together, they account for about two-thirds of all cells in a typical human body.

Physiological effects

The actions of insulin on the global human metabolism level include:

- Control of cellular intake of certain substances, most prominently glucose in muscle and adipose tissue (about two-thirds of body cells)

- Increase of DNA replication and protein synthesis via control of amino acid uptake

- Modification of the activity of numerous enzymes.

- The actions of insulin (indirect and direct) on cells include:

- Increased glycogen synthesis – insulin forces storage of glucose in liver (and muscle) cells in the form of glycogen; lowered levels of insulin cause liver cells to convert glycogen to glucose and excrete it into the blood. This is the clinical action of insulin, which is directly useful in reducing high blood glucose levels as in diabetes.

- Increased lipid synthesis – insulin forces fat cells to take in blood lipids, which are converted to triglycerides; lack of insulin causes the reverse

- Increased esterification of fatty acids – forces adipose tissue to make fats (i.e., triglycerides) from fatty acid esters; lack of insulin causes the reverse.

- Decreased proteolysis – decreasing the breakdown of protein

- Decreased lipolysis – forces reduction in conversion of fat cell lipid stores into blood fatty acids; lack of insulin causes the reverse.

- Decreased gluconeogenesis – decreases production of glucose from non-sugar substrates, primarily in the liver (the vast majority of endogenous insulin arriving at the liver never leaves the liver); lack of insulin causes glucose production from assorted substrates in the liver and elsewhere.

- Decreased autophagy - decreased level of degradation of damaged organelles. Postprandial levels inhibit autophagy completely.

- Increased amino acid uptake – forces cells to absorb circulating amino acids; lack of insulin inhibits absorption.

- Increased potassium uptake – forces cells to absorb serum potassium; lack of insulin inhibits absorption. Insulin's increase in cellular potassium uptake lowers potassium levels in blood.

- Arterial muscle tone – forces arterial wall muscle to relax, increasing blood flow, especially in micro arteries; lack of insulin reduces flow by allowing these muscles to contract.

- Increase in the secretion of hydrochloric acid by parietal cells in the stomach

- Decreased renal sodium excretion.

Insulin also influences other body functions, such as vascular compliance and cognition. Once insulin enters the human brain, it enhances learning and memory and benefits verbal memory in particular. Enhancing brain insulin signaling by means of intranasal insulin administration also enhances the acute thermoregulatory and glucoregulatory response to food intake, suggesting that central nervous insulin contributes to the control of whole-body energy homeostasis in humans.

Degradation.

Once an insulin molecule has docked onto the receptor and effected its action, it may be released back into the extracellular environment, or it may be degraded by the cell. The two primary sites for insulin clearance are the liver and the kidney. The liver clears most insulin during first-pass transit, whereas the kidney clears most of the insulin in systemic circulation. Degradation normally involves endocytosis of the insulin-receptor complex, followed by the action of insulin-degrading enzyme. An insulin molecule produced endogenously by the pancreatic beta cells is estimated to be degraded within about one hour after its initial release into circulation (insulin half-life ~ 4–6 minutes).

Hypoglycemia

Although other cells can use other fuels (most prominently fatty acids), neurons depend on glucose as a source of energy in the non-starving human. They do not require insulin to absorb glucose (unlike muscle and adipose tissue). They also have very small internal stores of glycogen. Glycogen stored in liver cells (unlike glycogen stored in muscle cells) can be converted to glucose, and released into the blood, when glucose from digestion is low or absent, and the glycerol backbone in triglycerides can also be used to produce blood glucose.

Sufficient lack of glucose and scarcity of these sources of glucose can dramatically make itself manifest in the impaired functioning of the central nervous system: dizziness, speech problems, and even loss of consciousness. Low blood glucose level is known as hypoglycemia or, in cases producing unconsciousness, "hypoglycemic coma" (sometimes termed "insulin shock" from the most common causative agent). Endogenous causes of insulin excess (such as an insulinoma) are very rare, and the overwhelming majority of insulin excess-induced hypoglycemia cases are accidentally caused by a physician's treatment. A few cases of murder, attempted murder, or suicide using insulin overdoses have been reported, but most insulin shocks appear to be due to errors in dosage of insulin (e.g., 20 units instead of 2) or other unanticipated factors (did not eat as much as anticipated, or exercised more than expected, or unpredicted kinetics of the subcutaneously injected insulin itself).

Possible causes of hypoglycemia include:

- External insulin (usually injected subcutaneously)

- Oral hypoglycemic agents (e.g., any of the sulfonylureas, or similar drugs, which increase insulin release from β-cells in response to a particular blood glucose level)

Ingestion of low-carbohydrate sugar substitutes in people without diabetes or with type 2 diabetes. Animal studies show these can trigger insulin release, albeit in much smaller quantities than sugar, according to a report in Discover magazine, August 2004, p 18. (This can never be a cause of hypoglycemia in patients with mature type 1 diabetes, since there is no endogenous insulin production to stimulate. It can occur during the honeymoon period, a period up to several years

after a type 1 diabetes diagnosis during which
endogenous insulin production still occurs.)

Part Four - Nutrition Details

Nutrition, exercise, and rest are the three pillars of health. If any one of them is lacking, then there is imbalance in the system. Imbalance causes sickness and disease.

Supplements

Everything a person needs can be acquired naturally with a good selection of food, water, fresh air, and some sunlight. Sometimes we use supplements because our schedule and daily nutrition intake are imperfect and therefore causing us to possibly suffer as a result of some nutritional deficiency.

Creatine plus Carbs

Creatine is a compound that is naturally made in our bodies to supply energy to our muscles. It is manufactured in the liver and may also be produced in the pancreas and kidneys. It is transported in the blood and taken up by muscle cells, where it is converted to creatine phosphate. The average person metabolizes about two grams of creatine per day, which happens to be about the same amount synthesized by the body. Thus, there is generally a balance maintained by the body. Once creatine is bound to a phosphate group, it is permanently stored in a cell as phosphocreatine until it is used to produce chemical energy called adenosine triphosphate (ATP). When this takes place, creatine can be released to form creatinine, which is then removed from the blood via the kidneys and excreted in the urine. Creatinine is routinely checked in blood tests, serving as a possible marker of how well the kidneys are filtering the blood. Although creatine supplementation can raise blood creatinine, it has never been shown to be toxic or harmful to the kidneys.

The most abundant natural source of creatine is in animal muscle, such as meats and fish. However, if one wishes to significantly boost athletic performance and make muscles grow large, then creatine must be taken in concentrations which are not easily obtained from a whole-food diet. For example, it would be necessary to eat ten pounds of raw steak per day for five days to successfully load the body with creatine.

Creatine supplements are used by athletes, bodybuilders, wrestlers, sprinters, and others who wish to gain muscle mass, typically consuming 2 to 3 times the amount that could be obtained from a very-high-protein diet. The Mayo Clinic states that creatine has been associated with asthmatic symptoms and warns against consumption by persons with known allergies to creatine.

There was once some concern that creatine supplementation could affect hydration status and heat tolerance and lead to muscle cramping and diarrhea, but recent studies have shown these concerns to be unfounded.

There are reports of kidney damage with creatine use, such as interstitial nephritis; patients with kidney disease should avoid use of this supplement. In similar manner, liver function may be altered, and caution is advised in those with underlying liver disease, although studies have shown little or no adverse impact on kidney or liver function from oral creatine supplementation. In 2004 the European Food Safety Authority (EFSA) published a record which stated that oral long-term intake of 3g pure creatine per day is risk-free. The reports of damage to the kidneys by creatine supplementation have been scientifically refuted.

Long-term administration of large quantities of creatine is reported to increase the production of formaldehyde, which has the potential to cause serious unwanted side-effects. However, this risk is largely theoretical because urinary excretion of formaldehyde, even under heavy creatine supplementation, does not exceed normal limits.

Extensive research has shown that oral creatine supplementation at a rate of 5 to 20 grams per day appears to be very safe and largely devoid of adverse side-effects, while at the same time effectively improving the physiological response to resistance exercise, increasing the maximal force production of muscles in both men and women.

A meta-analysis performed in 2008 found that creatine treatment resulted in no abnormal renal, hepatic, cardiac or muscle function.

Pharmacokinetics

Endogenous serum or plasma creatine concentrations in healthy adults are normally in a range of 2–12 mg/L. A single 5 g (5000 mg) oral dose in healthy adults results in a peak plasma creatine level of approximately 120 mg/L at 1–2 hours post-ingestion. Creatine has a fairly short elimination half-life, averaging just less than 3 hours, so to maintain an elevated plasma level it would be necessary to take small oral doses every 3–6 hours throughout the day. After the "loading dose" period

(1–2 weeks, 12-24 g a day), it is no longer necessary to maintain a consistently high serum level of creatine. As with most supplements, each person has their own genetic "preset" amount of creatine they can hold. The rest is eliminated out of the body as waste. Creatine is consumed by the body fairly quickly, and if one wishes to maintain the high concentration of creatine, Post-loading dose, 2-5 g daily is the standard amount to intake.

Pregnancy and breastfeeding

Creatine cannot be recommended during pregnancy or breastfeeding due to a lack of scientific information. Pasteurized cow's milk contains higher levels of creatine than human milk.

Treatment of diseases

Creatine has been demonstrated to cause modest increases in strength in people with a variety of neuromuscular disorders. Creatine supplementation has been, and continues to be, investigated as a possible therapeutic approach for the treatment of muscular, neuromuscular, neurological and neurodegenerative diseases, arthritis, congestive heart failure, Parkinson's disease, disuse atrophy, gyrate atrophy, McArdle's disease, Huntington's disease, miscellaneous neuromuscular diseases, mitochondrial diseases, muscular dystrophy, and neuro-protection, and depression.

A study demonstrated that creatine is twice as effective as the prescription drug riluzole in extending the lives of mice with the degenerative neural disease amyotrophic lateral sclerosis (ALS, or Lou Gehrig's disease). The neuro-protective effects of creatine in the mouse model of ALS may be due either to an increased availability of energy to injured nerve cells or to a blocking of the chemical pathway that leads to cell death. A similarly promising result has been obtained in prolonging the life of transgenic mice affected by Huntington's disease. Creatine treatment lessened brain atrophy and the formation of intra-nuclear inclusions, attenuated reductions in striatal N-acetyl-aspartate, and delayed the development of hyperglycemia.

Treatment of muscle disorders

A meta-analysis found that creatine treatment increased muscle strength in muscular dystrophies, and potentially improved functional performance. It has also been implicated in decreasing mutagenesis in DNA.

Improved cognitive ability

A placebo-controlled double-blind experiment found that a group of subjects composed of vegetarians and vegans who took 5 grams of creatine per day for six weeks showed a significant improvement on two separate tests of fluid intelligence, Raven's Progressive Matrices, and the backward digit span test from the WAIS. The treatment group was able to repeat longer sequences of numbers from memory and had higher overall IQ scores than the control group. The researchers concluded that "supplementation with creatine significantly increased intelligence compared with placebo. A subsequent study found that creatine supplements improved cognitive ability in the elderly. A study on young adults (0.03 g/kg/day for six weeks, e.g., 2 g/day for a 70-kilogram (150 lb) individual) failed to find any improvements.

Protein Shakes

What are protein shakes?

Protein is one of the body's main building blocks for muscle, bone, skin, and other tissues. Used often by athletes, protein shakes come in many combinations of protein, carbohydrates, and fats. They can range from 100% protein to mostly carbohydrates with a little added protein and fat. Protein shakes come in a variety of flavors in powder form or in ready-to-drink packages, such as cans or foil packs.

What are the benefits of protein shakes?

Safe for people who are healthy and fit, protein shakes are used mainly by athletes who need nourishment right after their workouts, says Jose Antonio, chief executive officer and co-founder of the International Society of Sports Nutrition (ISSN). 'Most people can't make a meal immediately post-workout', he says. 'So these ready-to-drink shakes are really your best alternative'.

According to the ISSN, protein shakes are a safe way to ensure enough protein, when used as part of a balanced, nutrient-rich diet. This counters the view that protein shakes can be harmful to kidneys or bones.

Although research hasn't proven their role in sports performance and muscle strength, protein shakes may offer certain benefits.

An endurance athlete may find it easier to train with the help of protein shakes, says Antonio. That's because they help the body recover from intense exercise. Protein shakes do this mainly by restoring muscle glycogen, a fuel source for exercise, which gets used up during workouts.

For the strength athlete, protein shakes can also help repair damage to muscles that can occur with serious bodybuilding.

The general fitness enthusiast who works out hard but doesn't want to be a marathon runner or bodybuilder may also benefit, says Antonio. This is the kind of person who might run twice a week and lift weights twice a week.

Some research shows other benefits as well. For example, a study of 130 U.S. Marines looked at intense exercisers who supplemented their diet with 10 g of protein, 8 g of carbohydrates, and 3 g of fat. They had fewer infections, less heat exhaustion, and less muscle soreness. Some protein shakes may help with weight management, as well. But more research is needed to confirm this.

How much protein do you need?

People get the protein they need from whole foods, milk, and protein drinks. The recommended daily intake of protein for healthy adults is 0.75 g of protein per pound of lean body weight.

The exact recommendations from Dr. Barry Sears, author of <u>The Zone</u> series of nutrition books is:

- 0.5 - Sedentary (no formal sports activity or training)
- 0.6 - Light Activity (ex. regular walking)
- 0.7 - Moderate Activity (3 days per week or sports participation)
- .08 - Active (Daily aerobic training or moderate weight training)
- 0.9 - Very Active (Intense weight training 3-4 days per week or other daily high volume exercise)
- - Elite Athlete(or weight training >5 days per week)

The formula is like this:

[? pounds – (? pounds X 0. ?)(estimated body fat percentage expressed as decimal)] X 0.75 = the number of grams of protein one should ingest

Let's say I weigh 180 pounds and I estimate myself at 15% body fat. The formula looks like this:

[180 - (180 X 0.15)] X 75 = 115 grams of protein

In most cases, only those who are active and restrict calories or are strict vegetarians are at risk for low protein.

People who exercise regularly need more energy. They may also need a little more protein than people who are less active. Adding protein doesn't add muscle. It simply gives the body enough protein to take care of business without having to cannibalize the muscles to get it.

What is the protein content of protein shakes?

Everyone, including athletes, can meet their protein needs without supplements or shakes. When choosing protein shakes, read the label to select the one with the composition that meets your needs.

Protein shakes vary in protein content. If you're a body builder, you're going to use the drinks that have more protein. Endurance athletes are should use drinks with more carbohydrates. The most important thing is to drink something with some nutrition after a workout.

If the goal is to lose body fat, change to a protein shake that's mainly protein, has fewer carbohydrates, and only a little bit of fat.

What are the different types of protein in protein shakes?

Protein shakes contain many different types of protein in varying amounts. They may include:

- Milk
- Whey
- Casein
- Egg
- Soy
- Rice

The source of the protein and how it's purified during manufacturing may affect how well the body can digest and absorb the amino acids, which are the building blocks of protein. Although it's best to obtain protein through diet, supplementing with a combination of whey and casein is a good way to quickly ingest some quickly digested nutrition, assuming you have no dairy allergies or intolerances.

Whey protein is:

- A protein found in milk
- Fast-absorbing
- In your body for a shorter time
- A good supplement after intense workouts

Casein protein is:

- The main protein in milk
- Slow-absorbing
- In your body for a longer time
- A good supplement for meal replacements or to take before bed

Soy protein is as effective as most animal sources of protein. Some women may take soy protein shakes in the hopes of curbing menopausal symptoms, but research results have been mixed.

Soy protein is:

- A plant-based source of protein
- As digestible as other sources of protein
- Known for its antioxidant capabilities
- A good supplement for meal replacements

Amino acids

Branched-chain amino acids are essential nutrients that the body obtains from proteins found in food, especially meat, dairy products, and legumes. "Branched-chain" refers to the chemical structure of these amino acids. People use branched-chain amino acids for medicine.

Branched-chain amino acids are used to treat:

- amyotrophic lateral sclerosis (ALS, Lou Gehrig's disease)
- brain conditions due to liver disease (chronic hepatic encephalopathy, latent hepatic encephalopathy)
- a movement disorder called tardive dyskinesia
- a genetic disease called McArdle's disease
- a disease called spinocerebellar degeneration
- Poor appetite in elderly kidney failure patients and cancer patients.

Branched-chain amino acids are also used to help slow muscle wasting in people who are confined to bed.

Some people use branched-chain amino acids to prevent fatigue and improve concentration.

Athletes use branched-chain amino acids to improve exercise performance and reduce protein and muscle breakdown during intense exercise.

Healthcare providers give branched-chain amino acids intravenously for sudden brain swelling due to liver disease (acute hepatic encephalopathy) and also when the body has been under extreme stress, for example after serious injury or widespread infection.

How does it work?

Branched-chain amino acids stimulate the building of protein in muscle and possibly reduce muscle breakdown. Branched-chain amino acids seem to prevent faulty message transmission in the brain cells of people with advanced liver disease, mania, tardive dyskinesia, and anorexia.

Glutamine

Glutamine is an amino acid (a building block for proteins), found naturally in the body.

Glutamine is used to counter some of the side effects of medical treatments. For example, it is used for side effects of cancer chemotherapy including diarrhea, pain and swelling inside the mouth (mucositis), nerve pain (neuropathy), and muscle and joint pains caused by the cancer drug Taxol. Glutamine is also used to protect the immune system and digestive system in people undergoing radiochemotherapy for cancer of the esophagus. Additionally, glutamine is used for improving recovery after bone marrow transplant or bowel surgery, increasing well-being in people who have suffered traumatic injuries, and preventing infections in critically ill people.

Some people use glutamine for digestive system conditions such as stomach ulcers, ulcerative colitis, and Crohn's disease. It is also used for depression, moodiness, irritability, anxiety, insomnia, and enhancing exercise performance.

People who have HIV (AIDS) sometimes use glutamine to prevent weight loss (HIV wasting).

Glutamine is also used for attention deficit-hyperactivity disorder (ADHD), a urinary condition called cystinuria, sickle cellanemia, and for alcohol withdrawal support.

Glutamine powder can be ordered through most wholesale drug suppliers. Glutamine for commercial use is made by a fermentation process using bacteria that produce glutamine.

How does it work?

Glutamine is the most abundant free amino acid in the body. Amino acids are the building blocks of protein. Glutamine is produced in the muscles and is distributed by the blood to the organs that need it. Glutamine might help gut function, the immune system, and other essential processes in the body, especially in times of stress. It is also important for providing "fuel" (nitrogen and carbon) to many different cells in the body. Glutamine is needed to make other chemicals in the body such as other amino acids and glucose (sugar).

After surgery or traumatic injury, nitrogen is necessary to repair the wounds and keep the vital organs functioning. About one third of this nitrogen comes from glutamine.

If the body uses more glutamine than the muscles can make (i.e., during times of stress), muscle wasting can occur. This can occur in people with HIV/AIDS. Taking glutamine supplements might keep the glutamine stores up.

Some types of chemotherapy can reduce the levels of glutamine in the body. Glutamine treatment is thought to help prevent chemotherapy-related damage by maintaining the life of the affected tissues.

Anti-Oxidants

"Free radicals" are unstable atoms, or molecules, in your body. They are missing important components that would make them more stable. So they rob other cells of those components to meet their needs. This causes injury to previously healthy cells. Over time, this damage can lead to diseases such as cancer, heart disease, or Alzheimer's disease.

Your body produces free radicals through its normal processes. Your body also contains antioxidant molecules, which deactivate harmful free radicals. But things like cigarette smoking, pollution, and excessive alcohol consumption can create so many free radicals that your body has a hard time defusing them on its own.

20 Common Foods With the Most Antioxidants

USDA scientists analyzed antioxidant levels in more than 100 different foods, including fruits and vegetables. Each food was measured for antioxidant concentration as well as antioxidant capacity per serving size. Cranberries, blueberries, and blackberries ranked highest among the fruits studied. Beans, artichokes, and Russet potatoes were tops among the vegetables. Pecans, walnuts, and hazelnuts ranked highest in the nut category. USDA chemist Ronald L. Prior says the total antioxidant capacity of the foods does not necessarily reflect their health benefit. Benefits depend on how the food's antioxidants are absorbed and utilized in the body. Still, this chart should help consumers trying to add more antioxidants to their daily diet.

k	Food item	Serving size	Total antioxidant capacity (per serving size)
1	Small Red Bean (dried)	Half cup	13,727
2	Wild blueberry	1 cup	13,427
3	Red kidney bean (dried)	Half cup	13,259
4	Pinto bean	Half cup	11,864
5	Blueberry (cultivated)	1 cup	9,019
6	Cranberry	1 cup (whole)	8,983
7	Artichoke (cooked)	1 cup (hearts)	7,904
8	Blackberry	1 cup	7,701
9	Prune	Half cup	7,291
10	Raspberry	1 cup	6,058
11	Strawberry	1 cup	5,938
12	Red Delicious apple	1 whole	5,900
13	Granny Smith apple	1 whole	5,381
14	Pecan	1 ounce	5,095
15	Sweet cherry	1 cup	4,873
16	Black plum	1 whole	4,844
17	Russet potato (cooked)	1 whole	4,649
18	Black bean (dried)	Half cup	4,181
19	Plum	1 whole	4,118
20	Gala apple	1 whole	3,903

Essential Fatty Acids

Omega-3 Fatty Acids: Fact Sheet

There are many health benefits of omega-3 fatty acids. Research shows strong evidence that the omega-3s EPA and DHA can help lower triglycerides and blood pressure. And there are studies showing that omega-3 fatty acids may help with other conditions, including rheumatoid arthritis, depression, and many more.

Just what are omega-3 fatty acids exactly? How much do you need? And what do all those abbreviations -- EPA, DHA, and ALA -- really mean? Here's a rundown on omega-3 fatty acids.

Omega-3 Fatty Acids: Basics

Omega-3 fatty acids are considered essential fatty acids. We need them for our bodies to work normally. Because essential fatty acids (ALA, DHA, EPA) are not made in the body or are inefficiently converted from ALA to EPA and DHA, we need to get them from our diet.

Omega-3s have a number of health benefits. Omega-3s are thought to play an important role in reducing inflammation throughout the body -- in the blood vessels, the joints, and elsewhere. However, omega-3 supplements (EPA/DHA) may cause the blood to thin and cause excess bleeding, particularly in people taking anticoagulant drugs.

There are several types of omega-3 fatty acids. Two crucial ones -- EPA and DHA -- are primarily found in certain fish. Plants like flax contain ALA, an omega-3 fatty acid that is partially converted into DHA and EPA in the body. Algae oil often provides only DHA.

Most experts say that DHA and EPA -- from fish and fish oil -- have better established health benefits than ALA. DHA and EPA are found together only in fatty fish and algae. DHA can also be found on its own in algae, while flaxseed and plant sources of omega-3s provide ALA -- a precursor to EPA and DHA, and a source of energy.

Omega-3 Fatty Acids: Benefits

Blood fat [triglycerides]. According to a number of studies, fish oil supplements can lower elevated triglyceride levels. Having high levels of this blood fat is a risk factor for heart disease. DHA alone has also been shown to lower triglycerides.

83

Rheumatoid arthritis. A number of studies have found that fish oil supplements [EPA+DHA] significantly reduced stiffness and joint pain. Omega-3 supplements also seem to boost the effectiveness of anti-inflammatory drugs.

Depression. Some researchers have found that cultures that eat foods with high levels of omega-3s have lower levels of depression. Fish oil also seems to boost the effects of antidepressants. Fish oil may help reduce the depressive symptoms of bipolar disorder.

Prenatal health. DHA appears to be important for visual and neurological development in infants. However, studies are inconclusive as to whether supplementing omega-3 during pregnancy or breastfeeding benefits the baby.

Asthma. Evidence suggests that a diet high in omega 3s reduces inflammation, a key component in asthma. However, more studies are needed to show if fish oil supplements improve lung function or reduce the amount of medication a person needs to control their disease.

ADHD. Some studies show that fish oil can reduce the symptoms of ADHD in some children and improve their cognitive function. However, more research is needed in this area, and omega-3 supplements as a primary treatment for this disorder are not supported by research.

Alzheimer's disease and dementia. The evidence is preliminary, but some research suggests that omega-3s may help protect against Alzheimer's disease and dementia. Recent studies have also evaluated whether the omega-3 supplement DHA can slow the decline seen in those with Alzheimer's dementia or in age-associated memory impairment. One recent study showed that DHA can be a beneficial supplement and may have a positive effect on gradual memory loss associated with aging. However, more research needs to be done.

Past evidence pointed to omega-3 fatty acids reducing risk of heart attacks, strokes and death from heart disease, but recent research has refuted these findings. More specific research is needed to sort this out.

Omega-3 Fatty Acids: Omega-3s and Omega-6s

You may have heard about the importance of having a healthy balance of omega-3s with another fatty acid, omega-6s. Omega-6s are found in many oils, meats, and processed foods. Some experts believe that most people in the U.S. are eating far too many omega-6s and far too few omega-3 fatty acids. They argue that this imbalance may be causing many chronic diseases. However, other experts disagree. They don't believe the ratio of omega-6s to omega-3s is actually significant. They also argue that the health benefits of omega-6s are being ignored. For now, the full implications aren't clear. But the bottom line is simple. Whether the ratio turns out to matter or not, increasing your intake of omega-3 fatty acids is still a good idea.

Omega-3 Fatty Acids: Food Sources

When possible, try to get omega-3 fatty acids from foods such as fish rather than supplements. Fish high in DHA and EPA omega-3 fatty acids include:

- anchovies
- bluefish
- herring
- mackerel
- salmon (wild has more omega-3s than farmed)
- sardines
- sturgeon
- lake trout

- tuna

Many experts recommend eating these fish two to three times a week.

Good food sources of ALA -- which is converted into omega-3 fatty acids in the body -- include:

- walnuts
- flax and flaxseed oil
- canola oil
- olive oil
- soybean oil

While foods containing omega-3 fatty acids have health benefits, some -- like oils and nuts -- can be high in calories. So eat them in moderation.

Omega-3 Fatty Acids: Supplements

If you decide to use a supplement, discuss this treatment with your doctor first to make sure you are getting the benefits you need. Experts usually recommend 1 gram (1,000 milligrams) of DHA and EPA combined from fish oil daily for those with heart disease. People with certain health conditions may take doses of up to 4 grams a day -- but only under a doctor's supervision.

The most common side effect from fish oil is indigestion and gas. Getting a supplement with an enteric coating might help.

Omega-3 supplements (EPA/DHA) can increase the risk of bleeding. People with bleeding conditions -- or who take medicines that could increase bleeding, like Coumadin, Plavix, Effient, Brilinta, and some nonsteroidal anti-inflammatory drugs -- should talk to a doctor before using any omega-3 supplements.

Omega-3 Fatty Acids: Tips

Choose the right fish. While eating more fatty fish is a good idea, some are more likely to have higher levels of mercury, PCBs, or other toxins. These include mackerel, wild swordfish, tilefish, and shark. Farm-raised fish of any type may also have higher levels of contaminants. Children and pregnant women should avoid these fish entirely. Everyone else should eat no more than 7 ounces of these fish a week. Smaller fish like wild trout and wild salmon are safer.

Consider a supplement like fish oil capsules or algae oil. Fish oil contains both EPA and DHA. Algae oil contains DHA and may be a good option for people who don't eat fish or for vegetarians.

Talk to your health care provider before using a supplement. Before you start using any supplement, you should always talk it over with your health care provider. He or she may have specific recommendations -- or warnings -- depending on your health and the other medicines you take.

Caffeine

Caffeine is a chemical found in coffee, tea, cola, guarana, mate, and other products.

Caffeine is most commonly used to improve mental alertness, but it has many other uses. Caffeine is used by mouth or rectally in combination with painkillers (such as aspirin and acetaminophen) and a chemical called ergotamine for treating migraine headaches. It is also used with painkillers for simple headaches and preventing and treating headaches after epidural anesthesia.

Some people use caffeine for asthma, gallbladder disease, attention deficit-hyperactivity disorder (ADHD), shortness of breath in newborns, and low blood pressure. Caffeine is also used for weight loss and type 2 diabetes. Very high doses are used, often in combination with ephedrine, as an alternative to illegal stimulants.

Caffeine is one of the most commonly used stimulants among athletes. Taking caffeine, within limits, is allowed by the National Collegiate Athletic Association (NCAA). Urine concentrations over 15 mcg/mL are prohibited. It takes most people about 8 cups of coffee providing 100 mg/cup to reach this urine concentration.

Caffeine creams are applied to the skin to reduce redness and itching in dermatitis.

Healthcare providers sometimes give caffeine intravenously (by IV) for headache after epidural anesthesia, breathing problems in newborns, and to increase urine flow.

In foods, caffeine is used as an ingredient in soft drinks, energy drinks, and other beverages.

People with voice disorders, singers, and other voice professionals are often advised against using caffeine. However, until recently, this recommendation was based only on hearsay. Now developing research seems to indicate that caffeine may actually harm voice quality. But further study is necessary to confirm these early findings.

How does it work?

Caffeine works by stimulating the central nervous system (CNS), heart, muscles, and the centers that control blood pressure. Caffeine can raise blood pressure, but might not have this effect in people who use it all the time. Caffeine can also act like a "water pill" that increases urine flow. But again, it may not have this effect in people who use caffeine regularly. Also, drinking caffeine during moderate exercise is not likely to cause dehydration.

Caffeine Myths and Facts

It's not always easy to know. Chances are you have some real misperceptions about caffeine. For starters, do you know the most common sources of caffeine? Well, maybe two of the sources aren't too hard to name -- coffee and tea leaves. But did you know kola nuts and cocoa beans are also included among the most common caffeine sources? And do you know how much caffeine content can vary from food to food? Turns out it's quite a lot actually, depending on the type and serving size of a food or beverage and how it's prepared.

Caffeine content can range from as much as 160 milligrams in some energy drinks to as little as 4 milligrams in a 1-ounce serving of chocolate-flavored syrup. Even decaffeinated coffee isn't completely free of caffeine. Caffeine is also present in some over-the-counter pain relievers, cold medications, and diet pills. These products can contain as little as 16 milligrams or as much as 200 milligrams of caffeine. In fact, caffeine itself is a mild painkiller and increases the effectiveness of other pain relievers.

Caffeine Myth No. 1: Caffeine Is Addictive

This one has some truth to it, depending on what you mean by "addictive." Caffeine is a stimulant to the central nervous system, and regular use of caffeine does cause mild physical dependence. But caffeine doesn't threaten your physical, social, or economic health the way addictive drugs do. (Although after seeing your monthly spending at the coffee shop, you might disagree!)

If you stop taking caffeine abruptly, you may have symptoms for a day or more, especially if you consume two or more cups of coffee a day. Symptoms of withdrawal from caffeine include:

- headache
- fatigue
- anxiety
- irritability

- depressed mood
- difficulty concentrating

No doubt, caffeine withdrawal can make for a few bad days. However, caffeine does not cause the severity of withdrawal or harmful drug-seeking behaviors as street drugs or alcohol. For this reason, most experts don't consider caffeine dependence a serious addiction.

Caffeine Myth No. 2: Caffeine Is Likely to Cause Insomnia

Your body quickly absorbs caffeine. But it also gets rid of it quickly. Processed mainly through the liver, caffeine has a relatively short half-life. This means it takes about five to seven hours, on average, to eliminate half of it from your body. After eight to 10 hours, 75% of the caffeine is gone. For most people, a cup of coffee or two in the morning won't interfere with sleep at night.

Consuming caffeine later in the day, however, can interfere with sleep. If you're like most people, your sleep won't be affected if you don't consume caffeine at least six hours before going to bed. Your sensitivity may vary, though, depending on your metabolism and the amount of caffeine you regularly consume. People who are more sensitive may not only experience insomnia but also have caffeine side effects of nervousness and gastrointestinal upset.

Caffeine Myth No. 3: Caffeine Increases the Risk of Osteoporosis, Heart Disease, and Cancer

Moderate amounts of daily caffeine -- about 300 milligrams, or three cups of coffee -- apparently cause no harm in most healthy adults. Some people are more vulnerable to its effects, however. That includes such people as those who have high blood pressure or are older. Here are the facts:

Osteoporosis and caffeine. At high levels (more than 744 milligrams/day), caffeine may increase calcium and magnesium loss in urine. But recent studies suggest it does not increase your risk for bone loss, especially if you get enough calcium. You can offset the calcium lost from drinking one cup of coffee by adding just two tablespoons of milk. However, research does show some links between caffeine and hip fracture risk in older adults. Older adults may be more sensitive to the effects of caffeine on calcium metabolism. If you're an older woman, discuss with your health care provider whether you should limit your daily caffeine intake to 300 milligrams or less.

Cardiovascular disease and caffeine. A slight, temporary rise in heart rate and blood pressure is common in those who are sensitive to caffeine. But several large studies do not link caffeine to higher cholesterol, irregular heartbeats, or an increased risk of cardiovascular disease. If you already have high blood pressure or heart problems, though, have a discussion with your doctor about your caffeine intake. You may be more sensitive to its effects. Also, more research is needed to tell whether caffeine increases the risk for stroke in people with high blood pressure.

Cancer and caffeine. Reviews of 13 studies involving 20,000 people revealed no relationship between cancer and caffeine. In fact, caffeine may even have a protective effect against certain cancers.

Caffeine Myth No. 4: Caffeine Is Harmful for Women Trying to Get Pregnant

Many studies show no links between low amounts of caffeine (a cup of coffee per day) and any of the following:

- trouble conceiving
- miscarriage
- birth defects

95

- premature birth
- low birth rate

At the same time, for pregnant women or those attempting pregnancy, the March of Dimes suggests fewer than 200 milligrams of caffeine per day. That's largely because in limited studies, women consuming higher amounts of caffeine had an increased risk for miscarriage.

Caffeine Myth No. 5: Caffeine Has a Dehydrating Effect

Caffeine can make you need to urinate. However, the fluid you consume in caffeinated beverages tends to offset the effects of fluid loss when you urinate. The bottom line is that although caffeine does act as a mild diuretic, studies show drinking caffeinated drinks in moderation doesn't actually cause dehydration.

Caffeine Myth No. 6: Caffeine Harms Children, Who, Today, Consume Even More Than Adults

As of 2004, children ages 6 to 9 consumed about 22 milligrams of caffeine per day. This is well within the recommended limit. However, energy drinks that contain a lot of caffeine are becoming increasingly popular, so this number may go up.

Some kids are sensitive to caffeine, developing temporary anxiety or irritability, with a "crash" afterwards. Also, most caffeine that kids drink is in sodas, energy drinks, or sweetened teas, all of which have high sugar content. These empty calories put kids at higher risk for obesity.

Even if the caffeine itself isn't harmful, caffeinated drinks are generally not good for kids.

Caffeine Myth No. 7: Caffeine Can Help You Sober Up

Actually, research suggests that people only think caffeine helps them sober up. For example, people who drink caffeine along with alcohol think they're OK behind the wheel. But the truth is reaction time and judgment are still impaired. College kids who drink both alcohol and caffeine are actually more likely to have car accidents.

Caffeine Myth No. 8: Caffeine Has No Health Benefits

Caffeine has few proven health benefits. But the list of caffeine's potential benefits is interesting. Any regular coffee drinker may tell you that caffeine improves alertness, concentration, energy, clear-headedness, and feelings of sociability. You might even be the type who needs that first cup o' Joe each morning before you say a single word. Scientific studies support these subjective findings. One French study even showed a slower decline in cognitive ability among women who consumed caffeine.

Other possible benefits include helping certain types of headache pain. Some people's asthma also appears to benefit from caffeine. These research findings are intriguing, but still need to be proven.

Limited evidence suggests caffeine may also reduce the risk of the following:

- Parkinson's disease
- liver disease
- colorectal cancer
- type 2 diabetes
- dementia

Despite its potential benefits, don't forget that high levels of caffeine may have adverse effects. More studies are needed to confirm both its benefits and potential risks.

Policicosanol: The Secret Cuban Sugar Cane Compound That Lowers Cholesterol

This information about policosanol comes from www.smart-publications.com. I learned about it from other sites when I my doctor insisted I start using statin drugs to treat some high cholesterol numbers. I asked about alternatives. He suggested we had nothing to talk about if I refused treatment. He is not my doctor today.

If you or someone you know has high cholesterol, you're probably familiar with the cholesterol-lowering drugs called "statins." Doctors hand them out like candy and sing their praises —because they work ... sort of.

In fact, in May 2001 when the National Institutes of Health issued the new cholesterol guidelines, doctors responded by saying that statins should be prescribed to some 36 million Americans, three times as many as the 13 million who had been taking them to reduce their risk of heart disease.

But besides their well-known side effects, (which you'll read about in this article), a new study suggests that statins also have subtle, insidious, far-reaching effects on the body ... that have the potential to unleash significant health problems down the road.

A Finnish study published in the Journal of American Medical Association February 2002 followed 120 men aged 35 to 64 years, who had high cholesterol that was previously untreated. The men were divided into two groups: one group continued with their usual diet and the other group ate a Mediterranean-style diet, including olive oil and fish (high in Omega-3 fatty acids), lots of fruits and vegetables, whole grains and low-fat proteins.

The groups were then subdivided, with one group from each of the original two groups taking either 20 mg of Simvastatin (Zocor) each day or a placebo. They followed this protocol for 12 weeks, and then each subgroup "crossed over" to the other treatment. There's no doubt about it. At the end of the 12-week study Zocor helped bring total cholesterol levels down 20.8 percent. In contrast, dietary intervention alone decreased total cholesterol by only 7.6 percent.[1]

But that's not all Zocor did. The drug also increased fasting serum insulin levels by 13 percent, and DECREASED serum concentrations of important antioxidant vitamins by as much as 22 percent! Also, the blood tests revealed significantly lower serum levels of critical nutrients like alpha-tocopherol, beta-carotene, and co-enzyme Q-10 while taking the statin drug, compared to the period when taking the placebo.1

This opens a whole new can of worms. Sure, the statin drug lowered the men's total cholesterol, but we're playing with very high stakes here, and the outcome is clearly a tradeoff. Zocor was found to lower levels of CoQ10, which is necessary for cardiovascular health, which means these men could very well end up with other heart health problems. And the 22 percent decrease in important antioxidants---well, we don't even want to comment on that! Because we all know how vital antioxidants are to our total health and protection against cancer, degenerative diseases, including Alzheimer's disease and arthritis, and cardiovascular disease! And the increase in insulin levels is a perfect set up for Syndrome X—which ultimately means weight gain leading to type 2 diabetes—one of the most dreaded diseases of our time—and other heart-health complications!

Diet and exercise certainly help, but if you or a loved one has high cholesterol, we want you know about

Policosanol. This new, natural product has been proven safer and more effective than statin drugs in dozens of studies. You can be assured you won't be suffering from any secondary illnesses down the road, or any of the common side effects associated with cholesterol-lowering drugs.

Policosanol: the new treatment for cholesterol management and reduced heart disease risk.

What is it?

Policosanol is a mixture of alcohols isolated and purified from sugar cane, whose main component is octacosanol. Policosanol has been studied extensively for the past 10 years and several human trials have been published in medical journals in North America and throughout the world. The clinical trials on humans have clearly demonstrated that Policosanol is safe, effective and without side effects.

Policosanol is actually not one thing, but a generic name for a highly concentrated and standardized mixture of five higher primary aliphatic alcohols that occur together naturally in sugar cane (Saccharum officinarum) wax. Although there are a few different forms of Policosanol (rice and beeswax), it is important to note that the results from the clinical trials were obtained using ONLY the Policosanol derived from sugar cane wax.

The studies on Policosanol are extremely impressive—and you'll see why. Most of them have been done in Cuba and since Cuban researchers are still working on getting the word out through scientific publications and peer-reviewed journals, Policosanol has yet to become a household word like statins—which is why we're so pleased to be at the forefront of bringing this information to you.

How does Policosanol work?

Because of the way that statin drugs work, they all have significant dose-related toxicity. If they inhibit the cholesterol-producing enzyme too much they can cause a variety of dangerous side effects. There is also growing concern among some scientists that statin drugs may have unknown long-term side effects, due to their mechanism of action in lowering cholesterol.

Amazingly, Policosanol has shown itself to be as effective as statin drugs for many of their varied beneficial effects WITHOUT showing any toxic effects. This is believed to be due to their different ways of helping control cholesterol levels. While statin drugs directly inhibit the cholesterol-producing enzyme, Policosanol instead seems to regulate the production of the enzyme to lower, more favorable levels.23 Policosanol also enhances our body's ability to remove and process LDL cholesterol from the blood and cells.4

Stops cardiovascular disease in its tracks

One of the most exciting effects of statin therapy is its ability to slow down or even reverse the progression of cardiovascular disease. This is often seen independent of the reduction in blood cholesterol levels. Research on Policosanol has provided evidence that it too can dramatically prevent, slow down, or even reverse the progression of cardiovascular disease.

Here are some highlights of the dozens of studies that have been published:

Cuban researchers found 5-20 mg daily of Policosanol to be effective at improving serum lipid profiles89 by:

- decreasing total cholesterol
- decreasing low-density lipoprotein (LDL), the "bad" cholesterol
- increasing high-density lipoprotein (HDL), the "good" cholesterol

- decreasing triglycerides

Policosanol was given to a large variety of patients with single health complaints and different combinations of disease. The outstanding common experience they all shared is this: ALL had improved lipid profiles after they took Policosanol.

Policosanol has been tested on:

- Healthy volunteers
- Patients with:
    - high cholesterol
    - type 2 diabetes
    - type 2 hypercholesterimia (an inherited genetic condition that results in elevated LDL levels beginning at birth, and possible heart attacks at an early age)
    - hypertension and high cholesterol
    - both high cholesterol and abnormal liver function tests
    - coronary patients
    - postmenopausal women with high cholesterol

German scientists amazed by results

A team of German scientists reviewed the literature on placebo-controlled lipid-lowering studies using Policosanol published in peer-reviewed journals as well as studies investigating its mechanism of action and its clinical pharmacology. This is what they found: At doses of 10 to 20 mg per day, Policosanol lowers total cholesterol by 17% to 21% and low-density lipoprotein (LDL) cholesterol by 21% to 29% and raises high-density lipoprotein cholesterol by 8% to 15%. {ref20}

Postmenopausal women have excellent results

When Policosonal was tested on postmenopausal women who had high cholesterol the results were equally impressive. 56 women were divided into two groups. One took a placebo and the other took 5mg of Policosanol for 8 weeks. For the second 8 weeks, the dosage was elevated to 10 mg of Policosanol.

Not only was Policosanol safe and well tolerated by the women, when it was compared to the women's baseline and the placebo group at both dosages of 5 and 10 mg a day it significantly:

- decreased LDL-cholesterol 17.3% and 26.7%, respectively
- decreased total cholesterol by 12.9% and 19.5%

- decreased the ratios of LDL-cholesterol to high-density lipoprotein (HDL)-cholesterol by 17.2% and 26.5%
- decreased total cholesterol to HDL-cholesterol by 16.3% and 21.0%
- raised HDL-cholesterol levels by 7.4% at the end of the study. No significant changes occurred in the lipid profile of the placebo group.21

Policosanol reduces blood lipids in older patients with type II hypercholesterolemia and high coronary risk

There's no doubt that patients with type II hypercholsterolemia (an inherited genetic condition that results in elevated LDL levels beginning at birth, and may result in heart attacks at an early age), have a very difficult time living without the fear of heart attack or stroke. In one Cuban study, after 6 weeks on a lipid-lowering diet, 179 older patients randomly received a placebo or Policosanol at doses of 5 mg followed by 10 mg per day for successive 12-week periods of each dose.

The results? Policosanol (5 and 10 mg/d):

- reduced low-density lipoprotein cholesterol by 16.9% and 24.4%, respectively

- reduced total cholesterol by 12.8% and 16.2%
- significantly increased high-density lipoprotein cholesterol (HDL) by 14.6% and 29.1%

Policosanol, but not the placebo, significantly improved overall cardiovascular health and stamina in these patients, and there were no adverse side effects!

Other studies which tested tolerability and effectiveness of Policosanol on patients with type II hypercholesterolaemia23, patients with hypertension and type II hypercholesterolaemia24, with hypercholesterolemia and noninsulin dependent diabetes, all had similar excellent results.

Policosanol outperforms most cholesterol-lowering drugs

In fact, Policosanol performed better than or equal to other cholesterol-lowering drugs, including Simvastatin, Pravastatin, Lovastatin, Probucol and Acipimox with fewer side effects.25 Daily doses of 10 mg of Policosanol have been shown to be equally effective in lowering total or LDL cholesterol as the same dose of simvastatin or pravastatin.2627

Is more effective than lovastatin in diabetics

Policosanol at 10 mg/day is more effective in normalizing HDL-cholesterol and has a better safety and tolerability profile than lovastatin at 20 mg/day in patients with high cholesterol and non-insulin dependent diabetes.[28]

Benefits beyond lowering cholesterol

Although scientists still don't know exactly how Policosanol works, study after study has shown it to decrease several other risk factors of cardiovascular disease:

- LDL oxidation[2930]
- platelet aggregation[3132]
- endothelial damage[33]

It also helps diminish the symptoms of intermittent claudication (peripheral arterial disease), a potentially disabling condition characterized by attacks of pain or fatigue in the calf, thigh or buttock.[34]

Treadmill test is easier with Policosanol!

If you're a heart patient, you've already endured the dreaded treadmill test. And if you've never taken it, you've probably heard about it. There was actually a study done following 45 heart patients with myocardial ischemia to see how Policosanol would affect their treadmill performance. The groups that took Policosanol for a 20-month period did significantly better on their treadmill tests than the group that took a placebo— due to an improvement in their myocardial ischemia—and also had improved lipid profiles.35

Proven safe!

Unlike statins, which become increasingly toxic with higher doses, Policosanol achieves its maximum effect at very low doses and taking more is neither more effective nor more toxic. In fact, Policosanol has undergone unusually extensive testing for a dietary supplement to prove its safety. Animal toxicity studies doses up to 1500 times the normal human dose (on the basis of body weight) have shown no negative effects on carcinogenesis3637 reproduction, growth, and development,3839 including a study on three generations of rats.

In studies where it has been given to animals (rats and dogs) in megadoses, no drug-related toxicity was shown, and there was no negative effect on the animals (including body weight gain, food consumption and blood biochemistry) when compared with the control group.414243

Prevention is the best cure

Abnormal cholesterol levels are one of the causes of atherosclerosis, which diminishes the supply of blood to the heart and eventually leads to heart attacks. Atherosclerosis affects blood vessels throughout your body and also contributes to angina (chest pain), intermittent claudication (pain caused by blockage of arteries in the legs), and stroke.

Do something about it before it's too late!

According to the guidelines set by the Expert Panel on Detection, Evaluation and Treatment of High Blood Cholesterol in Adults 44, the best things you can do for reducing heart disease is to:

- cut your intake of saturated fat and cholesterol
- reduce your consumption of carbohydrates
- exercise more
- control your weight

Vitamins

Vitamin A

The healthy eye needs to be able to deliver focused rays of visible light through various transparent media (cornea, crystalline lens, vitreous gel), so that those rays strike the retina and transmit a visual image to the brain.

Like other organs in the body, the eyes need a variety of specific nutrients in order to do their job. Vitamin A is critical to good vision. Vitamin A is a fat-soluble vitamin. That means it is absorbed into the bloodstream and stored in the liver, (the same is true for Vitamins D, E, and K). Vitamin A can be stored but those stores can also become depleted.

Vitamin A is essential for producing tears and keeping the surface of the eye moist and free of infection. Inadequate Vitamin A levels will also damage the clear cornea. Nearly everyone knows that carrots (loaded with Vitamin A) are healthy for the retinal cells – the photoreceptors. Poor vision in dim light (nyctalopia) is one of the earliest symptoms of Vitamin A deficiency, hypovitaminosis A. High-dose supplemental Vitamin A is prescribed as a treatment for some hereditary retinal disorders.

People tend to think of underserved Third World populations when the subject of malnutrition is discussed. It might surprise you to know that many Americans are malnourished, deficient in the key nutrients, minerals and vitamins essential for healthy living.

Malnourishment occurs in one of three situations: when a person fails to consume an adequate quantity of a necessary nutrient; when an individual's digestive tract cannot properly absorb the nutrition; or when a person's metabolism cannot correctly convert and store the digested products. Folks who have low Vitamin A levels can fit into each of these categories. I've got a few examples to share.

Patients who have undergone weight-loss surgery, like those popular gastric bypass procedures, are at risk of Vitamin A deficiency because their reconfigured anatomy short-circuits the absorption pathway. Anyone with liver problems is also at risk. Combine those people with the hordes who observe quirky exclusionary diets that deny the body of a healthy balance of vitamins and minerals. Your primary care doctor can help you determine if you are at risk.

Preserving your eyesight is a daily responsibility. Consuming a balanced diet rich in essential nutrients is an important part of maintaining healthy vision. It begins with Vitamin A.

Vitamin A is a nutrient that can be found in eggs, milk, liver, fortified cereals, carrots, spinach (and other leafy greens), and yellow or orange vegetables such as squash.

B Vitamins

The B vitamins, such as thiamine, riboflavin, B6, B12, and folic acid (folate) help the body with the health of red blood cells nerves, the heart, and the brain. Anemia, memory loss, fatigue, weakness, and digestive problems are signs of low B vitamins. These vitamins can be found in fish, meats, poultry, eggs, and dairy products.

Niacin (Vitamin B3)

Having enough niacin, or vitamin B3, in the body is important for general good health. As a treatment, higher amounts of niacin can improve cholesterol levels and lower cardiovascular risks.

Why do people take niacin?

As a cholesterol treatment, niacin has strong evidence. Several studies have shown that it can boost levels of good HDL cholesterol and lower triglycerides as well or better than some prescription drugs. Niacin also modestly lowers bad LDL cholesterol. It's often prescribed in combination with statins for cholesterol control, such as Crestor, Lescol, or Lipitor.

However, niacin is only effective as a cholesterol treatment at fairly high doses. These doses could pose risks, such as liver damage, gastrointestinal problems, or glucose intolerance. So don't treat yourself with over-the-counter niacin supplements. Instead, get advice from your health care provider, who can prescribe FDA-approved doses of niacin instead.

Niacin has other benefits. There's good evidence that it helps reduce atherosclerosis, or hardening of the arteries. For people who have already had a heart attack, niacin seems to lower the risk of a second one. In addition, niacin is an FDA-approved treatment for pellagra, a rare condition that develops from niacin deficiency.

Niacin has also been studied as a treatment for many other health problems. There's some evidence that it might help lower the risk of Alzheimer's disease, cataracts, osteoarthritis, and type 1 diabetes. However, more research needs to be done.

How much niacin should you take?

Since niacin can be used in different ways, talk to your health care provider about the best dosage for you.

Everyone needs a certain amount of niacin -- from food or supplements -- for the body to function normally. This amount is called the dietary reference intake (DRI), a term that is replacing the older and more familiar RDA (recommended daily allowance). For niacin, the DRIs vary with age and other factors.

- Children: between 2-16 milligrams daily, depending on age
- Men: 16 milligrams daily
- Women: 14 milligrams daily
- Women (pregnant): 18 milligrams daily
- Women (breastfeeding): 17 milligrams daily
- Maximum daily intake for adults of all ages: 35 milligrams daily

However, the ideal dosage of niacin depends on how you're using it. For instance, much higher doses -- 2 to 3 grams or more -- are used to treat high cholesterol.

Since niacin can upset your stomach, you might want to take it with food. To reduce flushing, your health care provider might recommend taking niacin along with aspirin, an NSAID painkiller, or an antihistamine for a few weeks until tolerance to the niacin develops.

Can you get niacin naturally from foods?

Niacin occurs naturally in many foods, including greens, meat, poultry, fish, and eggs, though in a fraction of the dose shown to achieve changes in cholesterol. Many products are also fortified with niacin during manufacture.

What are the risks of taking niacin?

Side effects. Niacin can cause flushing -- harmless but uncomfortable redness and warmth in the face and neck -- especially when you first begin taking it. Your health care provider will probably suggest increasing the dose slowly to reduce this problem. He or she might also offer a time-release prescription formulation to control flushing. Niacin can cause upset stomach and diarrhea. However, all of these side effects tend to fade over time.

Risks.

Niacin does have risks. It can cause liver problems, stomach ulcers, changes to glucose levels, muscle damage, low blood pressure, heart rhythm changes, and other issues. People with any health condition including liver or kidney disease, diabetes, high blood pressure, or cardiovascular problems need to talk to a doctor before using niacin supplements. Do not treat high cholesterol on your own with over-the-counter niacin supplements.

Interactions.

If you take any medicines or supplements regularly, talk to your doctor before you start using niacin supplements. They could interact with medicines like diabetes drugs, blood thinners, anticonvulsants, blood pressure medicines, thyroid hormones, and antibiotics as well as supplements like ginkgo biloba and some antioxidants. Alcohol might increase the risk of liver problems. Though niacin is often used along with statins for high cholesterol, this combination may increase the risk for side effects. Get advice from your health care provider.

At the low DRI doses, niacin is safe for everyone. However, at the higher amounts used to treat medical conditions, it can have risks. For that reason, children and women who are pregnant or breastfeeding should not take niacin supplements in excess of the DRI unless it's recommended by a doctor.

Vitamin B-12 (Cobalamin)

Vitamin B-12 (cobalamin) plays a role in making DNA. Vitamin B-12 also helps keep nerve cells and red blood cells healthy.

Why do people take vitamin B-12?

Vitamin B-12 has been looked at as a treatment for many diseases and conditions. These include fatigue, Alzheimer's disease, heart disease, breast cancer, high cholesterol, and sickle cell disease. However, the results have been inconclusive. Studies suggest that vitamin B-12 does not help with stroke risk or lung cancer.

Vitamin B-12 supplements do help people who have a deficiency. Low levels of vitamin B-12 are more likely in people over 50. Vitamin B-12 is also more common in those with certain conditions, like digestive problems and some types of anemia. Low vitamin B-12 can cause fatigue, weakness, memory loss, and other problems with the nervous system.

There is some conflicting evidence about using vitamin B-12 to treat elevated levels of homocysteine in the blood. It is not fully understood how or if this elevation contributes to heart disease and other problems with blood vessels, or if the elevation is a result of these conditions. A high level of homocysteine in the blood is a risk factor for coronary, cerebral, and peripheral blood vessel disease. Risks also include blood clots, heart attacks, and certain types of stroke.

Since the evidence for treating elevated levels of homocysteine in the blood remains conflicting, the current recommendation is screening of men over 40 and women over 50. For patients with elevated homocysteine levels, the recommendation is to supplement with folic acid and vitamin B-12. You should talk to your doctor before treating yourself for these conditions.

A recent study showed that vitamin B-12, used with folic acid and vitamin B6, reduces the risk for age-related macular degeneration (AMD) in women with heart disease or multiple risk factors for heart disease.

How much vitamin B-12 should you take?

The recommended dietary allowance (RDA) includes the vitamin B-12 you get from both food and any supplements you take.

Vitamin B-12: Recommended Dietary Allowance (RDA) in micrograms (mcg)

- 0-6 months - 0.4 micrograms/day
- 7-12 months - 0.5 mcg/day
- 1-3 years - 0.9 mcg/day
- 4-8 years - 1.2 mcg/day
- 9-13 years - 1.8 mcg/day
- 14 years and up - 2.4 mcg/day
- Pregnant women - 2.6 mcg/day
- Breastfeeding women - 2.8 mcg/day

Even at high doses, vitamin B-12 seems fairly safe. Experts have not found a specific dose of vitamin B-12 that's dangerous. No tolerable upper intake levels have been set.

Can you get vitamin B-12 naturally from foods?

Some good food sources of vitamin B-12 are:

- Fish and shellfish
- Meats
- Poultry and eggs
- Dairy products
- Fortified cereals

Generally, it's best to get vitamins from whole foods. But doctors often suggest fortified foods -- and supplements -- to people over 50. As we age, it's harder for our bodies to absorb vitamin B-12 from food.

What are the risks of taking vitamin B-12?

Side effects and risks. Taken at normal doses, side effects are rare. High doses may cause acne. Allergies to vitamin B-12 supplements have been reported and can cause swelling, itchy skin, and shock.

Interactions. Drugs for acid reflux, diabetes, and other conditions may make it harder for your body to absorb vitamin B-12.

Vitamin C

Vitamin C is one of the safest and most effective nutrients, experts say. It may not be the cure for the common cold (though it's thought to help prevent more serious complications). But the benefits of vitamin C may include protection against immune system deficiencies, cardiovascular disease, prenatal health problems, eye disease, and even skin wrinkling.

A recent study published in Seminars in Preventive and Alternative Medicine that looked at over 100 studies over 10 years revealed a growing list of benefits of vitamin C.

"Vitamin C has received a great deal of attention, and with good reason. Higher blood levels of vitamin C may be the ideal nutrition marker for overall health," says study researcher Mark Moyad, MD, MPH, of the University of Michigan. "The more we study vitamin C, the better our understanding of how diverse it is in protecting our health, from cardiovascular, cancer, stroke, eye health [and] immunity to living longer."

"But," Moyad notes, "the ideal dosage may be higher than the recommended dietary allowance."

How Much Vitamin C Is Enough?

Most of the studies Moyad and his colleagues examined used 500 daily milligrams of vitamin C to achieve health results. That's much higher than the RDA of 75-90 milligrams a day for adults. So unless you can eat plenty of fruits and vegetables, you may need to take a dietary supplement of vitamin C to gain all the benefits, Moyad says. He suggests taking 500 milligrams a day, in addition to eating five servings of fruits and vegetables.

"It is just not practical for most people to consume the required servings of fruits and vegetables needed on a consistent basis, whereas taking a once-daily supplement is safe, effective, and easy to do," Moyad says. He also notes that only 10% to 20% of adults get the recommended nine servings of fruits and vegetables daily.

Moyad says there is no real downside to taking a 500-milligram supplement, except that some types may irritate the stomach. That's why he recommends taking a non-acidic, buffered form of the vitamin. "The safe upper limit for vitamin C is 2,000 milligrams a day, and there is a great track record with strong evidence that taking 500 milligrams daily is safe," he says.

Still, American Dietetic Association spokeswoman Dee Sandquist, RD, suggests doing your best to work more fruits and vegetables into your diet before taking supplements.

"Strive to eat nine servings of fruits and vegetables daily, because you will get a healthy dose of vitamin C along with an abundance of other vitamins, minerals, and phytochemicals that are good for disease prevention and overall health," she says.

While a cup of orange juice or a half-cup of red pepper would be enough to meet your RDA for Vitamin C, here are all the foods and beverages you'd need to consume to reach 500 milligrams (mg):

- Cantaloupe, 1 cup (8 ounces): 59mg
- Orange juice, 1 cup: 97mg
- Broccoli, cooked, 1 cup: 74mg
- Red cabbage, 1/2 cup: 40mg
- Green pepper, 1/2 cup, 60mg
- Red pepper, 1/2 cup, 95mg
- Kiwi, 1 medium: 70mg
- Tomato juice, 1 cup: 45mg.

According to recent research, vitamin C may offer health benefits in these areas:

1. Stress. "A recent meta-analysis showed vitamin C was beneficial to individuals whose immune system was weakened due to stress -- a condition which is very common in our society," says Moyad. And, he adds, "because vitamin C is one of the nutrients sensitive to stress, and [is] the first nutrient to be depleted in alcoholics, smokers, and obese individuals, it makes it an ideal marker for overall health."

2. Colds. When it comes to the common cold, vitamin C may not be a cure. But some studies show that it may help prevent more serious complications. "There is good evidence taking vitamin C for colds and flu can reduce the risk of developing further complications, such as pneumonia and lung infections," says Moyad.

3. Stroke. Although research has been conflicting, one study in the American Journal of Clinical Nutrition found that those with the highest concentrations of vitamin C in their blood were associated with 42% lower stroke risk than those with the lowest concentrations. The reasons for this are not completely clear. But what is clear is that people who eat plenty of fruits and

vegetables have higher blood levels of vitamin C.

"People who consume more fruit and vegetables will not only have higher [blood] levels of vitamin C, but higher intake of other nutrients potentially beneficial to health, such as fiber and other vitamins and minerals," study researcher Phyo K. Myint said in an email interview.

4. Skin Aging. Vitamin C affects cells on the inside and outside of the body. A study published in the American Journal of Clinical Nutrition examined links between nutrient intakes and skin aging in 4,025 women aged 40-74. It found that higher vitamin C intakes were associated with a lower likelihood of a wrinkled appearance, dryness of the skin, and a better skin-aging appearance.

Other studies have suggested that vitamin C may also:

- Improve macular degeneration.
- Reduce inflammation.
- Reduce the risk of cancer and cardiovascular disease.

Vitamin C's Role in the Body

Vitamin C, also known as ascorbic acid, is necessary for the growth, development and repair of all body tissues. It's involved in many body functions, including formation of collagen, absorption of iron, the immune system, wound healing, and the maintenance of cartilage, bones, and teeth.

Vitamin C is one of many antioxidants that can protect against damage caused by harmful molecules called free radicals, as well as toxic chemicals and pollutants like cigarette smoke. Free radicals can build up and contribute to the development of health conditions such as cancer, heart disease, and arthritis.

Vitamin C is not stored in the body (excess amounts are excreted), so overdose is not a concern. But it's still important not to exceed the safe upper limit of 2,000 milligrams a day to avoid stomach upset and diarrhea.

Water-soluble vitamins must be continuously supplied in the diet to maintain healthy levels. Eat vitamin-C-rich fruits and vegetables raw, or cook them with minimal water so you don't lose some of the water-soluble vitamin in the cooking water.

Vitamin C is easily absorbed both in food and in pill form, and it can enhance the absorption of iron when the two are eaten together.

Deficiency of vitamin C is relatively rare, and primarily seen in malnourished adults. In extreme cases, it can lead to scurvy -- characterized by weakness, anemia, bruising, bleeding, and loose teeth.

How to Get More Vitamin C in Your Diet

This antioxidant super-nutrient is found in a variety of fruits and vegetables. Yet, according to dietary intake data and the 2005 U.S. Dietary Guidelines, most adults don't get enough vitamin C in their diets. This is especially true of smokers and non-Hispanic black males, according to research done by Jeff Hampl, PhD, RD, and colleagues at the University of Arizona.

The foods richest in vitamin C are citrus fruits, green peppers, strawberries, tomatoes, broccoli, white potatoes, and sweet potatoes. Other good sources include dark leafy greens, cantaloupe, papaya, mango, watermelon, brussels sprouts, cauliflower, cabbage, red peppers, raspberries, blueberries, winter squash, and pineapples.

Vitamin D

Vitamin D plays several key roles in your body. Most importantly, vitamin D helps your body absorb the minerals calcium and phosphorus from the food you eat, which is important for bone health.

Many Americans have been found to have low levels of vitamin D. The reasons for this include low availability of vitamin D in food sources, increased time working indoors, and possibly increased use of sunscreens (since sunlight helps the body produce vitamin D).

Certain people may benefit from vitamin D supplementation. However, there is conflicting evidence about the amount of vitamin D that is safe and effective, or even necessary, to use as a supplement.

Why do people take vitamin D?

Vitamin D is important for people with osteoporosis. Studies show that calcium and vitamin D together can increase bone density in postmenopausal women. Vitamin D also helps with other disorders associated with weak bones, like rickets.

People who have low levels of vitamin D may need supplements. Vitamin D deficiencies are more common in those who:

- Are over 50
- Get very little sun exposure
- Have kidney disease or diseases that affect the absorption of minerals
- Have darker skin
- Are lactose intolerant
- Are vegan
- Are infants who are fed only breast milk

Vitamin D deficiency is commonly seen in people living in the Northern parts of the U.S.

Vitamin D deficiency may cause hormone problems, muscle weakness and pain, and other symptoms.

Studies have found prescription-strength vitamin D lotions helpful in treating psoriasis. Vitamin D has also been studied for other conditions ranging from cancer prevention to high blood pressure, but the evidence is unclear.

How much vitamin D should you take?

The Institute of Medicine (IOM) has set a recommended dietary allowance for vitamin D. Getting this amount of vitamin D from diet, with or

131

without supplements, should be enough to keep you healthy.

- 600 IU/day for anyone aged 1-70
- 800 IU/day for anyone over 70

Some experts think that these recommendations are too low, especially for people at risk of osteoporosis. Ask your health care provider how much vitamin D you need.

Recently the IOM reviewed more than 1,000 research papers on vitamin D and concluded that high levels of the supplement are unnecessary and could be harmful.

The IOM warned that doses above 4,000 units a day were potentially harmful and that doses above 10,000 IU per day are associated with kidney and tissue damage.

Can you get vitamin D naturally from foods?

The best source of natural vitamin D is sunlight. Just 10 to 15 minutes of exposure without sunscreen a couple of times a week usually gives you enough vitamin D.

Vitamin D is also naturally found in butter, eggs, and fish such as salmon, tuna and mackerel. Vitamin D is often added to fortified foods, too, such as milk and cereal.

What are the risks of taking vitamin D?

Side effects. At normal doses, vitamin D seems to have few side effects.

Interactions. Vitamin D can interact with many medicines, such as drugs for high blood pressure and heart problems. If you take daily medicine, ask your health care provider if it's safe for you to take vitamin D supplements.

Risks. Too much vitamin D can cause loss of appetite, frequent urination, and weight loss. High doses of vitamin D can also lead to disorientation and kidney and heart problems.

Vitamin E

Vitamin E is key for strong immunity and healthy skin and eyes. In recent years, vitamin E supplements have become popular as antioxidants. These are substances that protect cells from damage. However, the risks and benefits of taking vitamin E supplements are still unclear.

Why do people take vitamin E?

Many people use vitamin E supplements in the hopes that the vitamin's antioxidant properties will prevent or treat disease. But studies of vitamin E for preventing cancer, heart disease, diabetes, Alzheimer's disease, cataracts, and many other conditions have been inconclusive.

So far, the only established benefits of vitamin E supplements are in people who have an actual deficiency. Vitamin E deficiencies are rare. They're more likely in people who have diseases, such as digestive problems and cystic fibrosis. People on very low-fat diets may also have low levels of vitamin E.

How much vitamin E should you take?

The recommended dietary allowance (RDA) includes the vitamin E you get from both the food you eat and any supplements you take.

Vitamin E (alpha-tocopherol): Recommended Dietary Allowance (RDA)

CHILDREN

- 1-3 years - 6 mg/day (9 IU)
- 4-8 years - 7 mg/day (10.4 IU)

- 9-13 years - 11 mg/day (16.4 IU)

FEMALES

- 14 years and up - 15 mg/day (22.4 IU)
- Pregnant - 15 mg/day (22.4 IU)
- Breastfeeding - 19 mg/day (28.5 IU)

MALES

- 14 years and up - 15 mg/day (22.4 IU)

The tolerable upper intake levels of a supplement are the highest amount that most people can take safely. Higher doses might be used to treat vitamin E deficiencies. But you should never take more unless a doctor says so.

Tolerable Upper Intake Levels (UL) of Vitamin E (alpha-tocopherol)

- 1-3 years - 200 mg/day (300 IU)
- 4-8 years - 300 mg/day (450 IU)
- 9-13 years - 600 mg/day (900 IU)
- 14-18 years - 800 mg/day (1,200 IU)
- 19 years and up - 1,000 mg/day (1,500 IU)

Because vitamin E is fat-soluble, supplements are best absorbed with food.

Can you get vitamin E naturally from foods?

Most people get enough vitamin E from food. Good sources of vitamin E include:

- Vegetable oils
- Green leafy vegetables, like spinach
- Fortified cereals and other foods
- Eggs
- Nuts

What are the risks of taking vitamin E?

The risks and benefits of taking vitamin E are still unclear. Long-term use (over 10 years) of vitamin E has been linked to an increase in stroke.

In addition, an analysis of clinical trials found patients who took either synthetic vitamin E or natural vitamin E in doses of 400 IU per day -- or higher -- had an increased risk of dying from all causes, which seems to increase even more at higher doses. Cardiovascular studies also suggest that patients with diabetes or cardiovascular disease who take natural vitamin E at 400 IU per day have an increased risk of heart failure and heart failure-related hospitalization.

Vitamin E supplements might be harmful when taken in early pregnancy. One study found that women who took vitamin E supplementation during the first 8 weeks of pregnancy had a 1.7 to nine-fold increase in congenital heart defects. The exact amount of vitamin E supplements used by pregnant women in this study is unknown.

A large population study showed that men using a multivitamin more than seven times per week in conjunction with a separate vitamin E supplement actually had a significantly increased risk of developing prostate cancer.

The American Heart Association recommends obtaining antioxidants, including vitamin E, by eating a well-balanced diet high in fruits, vegetables, and whole grains rather than from supplements. If you are considering taking a vitamin E supplement, talk to your health care provider first to see if it is right for you.

What are the side effects of taking vitamin E?

Topical vitamin E can irritate the skin.

Overdoses of vitamin E supplements can cause nausea, headache, bleeding, fatigue, and other symptoms. It can also cause kidney failure.

People who take blood thinners or other medicines should not take vitamin E supplements without first talking to their health care provider.

Vitamin K

Vitamin K is a vitamin found in leafy green vegetables, broccoli, and Brussels sprouts. The name vitamin K comes from the German word "Koagulationsvitamin."

Several forms of vitamin K are used around the world as medicine. But in the U.S., the only form available is vitamin K1 (phytonadione). Vitamin K1 is generally the preferred form of vitamin K because it is less toxic, works faster, is stronger, and works better for certain conditions.

In the body, vitamin K plays a major role in blood clotting. So it is used to reverse the effects of "blood thinning" medications when too much is given; to prevent clotting problems in newborns who don't have enough vitamin K; and to treat bleeding caused by medications including salicylates, sulfonamides, quinine, quinidine, or antibiotics. Vitamin K is also given to treat and prevent vitamin K deficiency, a condition in which the body doesn't have enough vitamin K. It is also used to prevent and treat weak bones (osteoporosis) and relieve itching that often accompanies a liver disease called biliary cirrhosis.

People apply vitamin K to the skin to remove spider veins, bruises, scars, stretch marks, and burns. It is also used topically to treat rosacea, a skin condition that causes redness and pimples on the face. After surgery, vitamin K is used to speed up skin healing and reduce bruising and swelling.

Healthcare providers also give vitamin K by injection to treat clotting problems.

An increased understanding of the role of vitamin K in the body beyond blood clotting led some researchers to suggest that the recommended amounts for dietary intake of vitamin K be increased. In 2001, the National Institute of Medicine Food and Nutrition Board increased their recommended amounts of vitamin K slightly, but refused to make larger increases. They explained there wasn't enough scientific evidence to make larger increases in the recommended amount of vitamin K.

How does it work?

Vitamin K is an essential vitamin that is needed by the body for blood clotting and other important processes.

Minerals

Calcium

You've heard that calcium protects your bones and that your milk glass is loaded with it -- but what do you really know about this essential nutrient? Most people may not realize that calcium is the most abundant mineral in the body. Or that calcium does far more than just strengthen your bones and teeth.

Here's a quick primer on calcium -- including why you need it and where to get it.

Calcium is probably best known for strengthening bones and teeth. In fact, most of the calcium in our bodies is stored in the bones and teeth. As bones undergo their regular process of breakdown and remodeling, calcium helps build new bone.

Getting enough calcium is important for keeping your bones strong throughout your lifetime, but especially during childhood, while the bones are still growing. It's also essential during the senior years, when bones start to break down faster than they can rebuild. Older bones become more brittle and easily fractured -- a condition called osteoporosis.

- Calcium also plays an important role in several other body functions, including:
- Nerve signal transmission
- Hormone release
- Muscle contraction
- Blood vessel function
- Blood clotting

There's also some early evidence that calcium might lower blood pressure and help protect against colorectal and prostate cancers. However, these benefits have yet to be confirmed in studies.

How Much Calcium Do You Need?

How much calcium you need depends on your age and gender. The recommended daily dietary allowances for calcium are:

Age	Male	Female
1-3 years	700 mg	700 mg
4-8 years	1,000 mg	1,000 mg
9-13 years	1,300 mg	1,300 mg
14-18 years	1,300 mg	1,300 mg
19-50 years	1,000 mg	1,000 mg

- 51-70 years   1,000 mg   1,200 mg
- 71+ years   1,200 mg   1,200 mg

Getting much more than the recommended amount of calcium from food and supplements increases the risk of side effects, so it's best to avoid taking too much.

Where Should You Get Calcium?

The ideal way to get calcium is from foods. Dairy products such as milk, cheese, and yogurt are the obvious sources. One 8-ounce cup of low-fat, plain yogurt contains 415 mg of calcium -- more than a third of the daily recommendation for most age groups. An 8-ounce glass of nonfat milk will provide you nearly 300 mg of calcium. And 1.5 ounces of part-skim mozzarella has 333 mg.

Even if you're lactose intolerant, you can still enjoy your milk by choosing one of the lactose-free or lactose-reduced dairy products available at your local supermarket. Another option is to take lactase enzyme drops or tablets before you eat dairy.

Several non-dairy foods are also good sources of calcium, including:

- Food Item   Calcium content per serving
- Calcium-fortified orange juice, 6 ounces 375 mg
- Canned sardines with bones, 3 ounces 325 mg
- Firm tofu made with calcium sulfate, 1/2 cup 253 mg
- Canned salmon with bone, 3 ounces 181 mg
- Calcium-fortified breakfast cereal, 1 cup 100-1,000 mg
- Boiled turnip greens, 1/2 cup 99 mg
- Cooked fresh kale, 1 cup 94 mg

Taking Calcium Supplements

If you're not getting enough calcium from food alone, your doctor might recommend a supplement.

Calcium supplements come in two main forms:

- Calcium carbonate -- found in products such as Caltrate 600, Os-Cal 500, Viactiv Calcium Chews, and store brands

- Calcium citrate -- found in supplements such as Citracal

Calcium carbonate is also commonly found in over-the-counter antacids, such as Rolaids and Tums.

You need to take calcium carbonate with food, because it's easier for your body to absorb that way. You can take calcium citrate on an empty stomach.

To maximize your absorption of calcium, take no more than 500 mg at a time. You might take one 500-mg supplement in the morning and another at night. If you take a supplement that also contains vitamin D, it will help your body absorb calcium more efficiently.

Avoid eating these foods when you take your supplement, because they can interfere with calcium absorption:

- Caffeinated coffee and soda
- High-salt foods

Calcium Supplement Side Effects

Before taking calcium supplements, you need to be aware of their side effects, which include:

- Constipation
- Gas or bloating
- Kidney stones

Calcium can also decrease absorption of some medicines, including osteoporosis medicines, thyroid medicines, and some antibiotics. Ask your doctor if your medicines may interact with calcium, or to be safe just don't take them at the same time. Taking calcium and vitamin D supplements with thiazide diuretics may increase the chance of kidney stones.

A June 2012 study in the journal Heart also linked calcium supplements with a greater likelihood of heart attacks. This finding may be of special concern to anyone who is already at risk for heart disease.

Experts disagree regarding who should take calcium and vitamin D supplements. The U.S. Preventive Services Task Force doesn't recommend taking calcium supplements to prevent osteoporosis-related fractures in postmenopausal women because the organization says there isn't enough evidence to support a benefit. Other organizations, including the National Osteoporosis Foundation and the Institute of Medicine, recommend supplements if you're not meeting your daily calcium requirements with diet alone.

Although your bones need calcium, don't take any supplements without first talking to your doctor. Find out which form of calcium is best for you to take, how much you need each day, and what to do if you experience any side effects.

Iron

Iron is a mineral that's necessary for life. Iron plays a key role in the making of red blood cells, which carry oxygen. You can get iron from food and from supplements. If you don't have enough iron, you may develop anemia, a low level of red blood cells.

Why do people take iron?

Iron supplements are most often used for certain types of anemia. Anemia can cause fatigue and other symptoms. If you have symptoms of anemia, seek care from your health care provider. Don't try to treat it on your own.

Iron supplements are often used to treat anemia caused by:

- Pregnancy
- Heavy menstrual periods

- Kidney disease
- Chemotherapy

Iron supplements have also been studied for treatment of ADHD. While early data suggested a benefit, more study is needed before iron can be recommended for ADHD.

Iron supplements are commonly recommended for infants and toddlers, teenage girls, and women who are pregnant or of childbearing age to help prevent anemia. Before taking an iron supplement, ask your health care provider if it is right for you.

How much iron should you take?

The recommended dietary allowance (RDA) includes the iron you get from both the food you eat and any supplements you take.

CHILDREN

- 7-12 months - 11 mg/day
- 1-3 years - 7 mg/day
- 4-8 years - 10 mg/day
- 9-13 years - 8 mg/day

FEMALES

- 14-18 years - 15 mg/day
- 19-50 years - 18 mg/day

- 51 years and over - 8 mg/day
- Pregnant - 27 mg/day

Breastfeeding

- Under 19 years: 10 mg/day
- 19 years and over: 9 mg/day

MALES

- 14-18 years - 11 mg/day
- 19 years and up - 8 mg/day

Take iron supplements with a full glass of water or food. Strict vegetarians may need to take in higher levels of iron.

At high doses, iron is toxic. For adults and children ages 14 and up, the upper limit -- the highest dose that can be taken safely -- is 45 mg a day. Children under 14 should not take more than 40 mg a day.

The American Academy of Pediatrics suggests that -- starting at 4 months of age -- breastfed infants should be supplemented with 1 mg/kg per day of oral iron. This should continue until iron-containing complementary foods, such as iron-fortified cereals, are introduced in the diet.

Also beginning at 4 months of age, partially breastfed infants (more than half of their daily feedings as formula or milk) who are not receiving iron-containing complementary foods should receive 1 mg/kg per day of supplemental iron.

Ask your health care provider how much iron supplement you or your child should take, if any.

Can you get iron naturally from foods?

For most people, a good diet provides enough iron. Natural food sources of iron include:

- Meat, fish, and poultry
- Vegetables, like spinach, kale, and broccoli
- Dried fruits and nuts
- Beans, lentils, and peas

Iron is also added to many fortified foods, such as cereals and enriched breads.

What are the risks of taking iron?

Side effects. Taken at normal doses, iron supplements may cause upset stomach, stool changes, and constipation.

Risks. Don't start taking iron supplements unless your health care provider tells you that you need them. That's especially true if you have a chronic health condition. Women who plan to become pregnant should also check with a health care provider before they start daily iron supplements.

Interactions. Iron can interact with many different drugs and supplements. They include antacids, anti-inflammatory painkillers, antibiotics, calcium, and others. If you take daily medicine, ask your health care provider if it's safe for you to take iron supplements.

Overdose. Iron overdose is a common cause of poisoning in children. It can be fatal. Signs of an iron overdose include severe vomiting and diarrhea, stomach cramps, pale or bluish skin and fingernails, and weakness. Treat these signs as a medical emergency. Call poison control and get medical help immediately.

Manganese

Manganese is a mineral that is found in several foods including nuts, legumes, seeds, tea, whole grains, and leafy green vegetables. It is considered an essential nutrient, because the body requires it to function properly. People use manganese as medicine.
Manganese is used for prevention and treatment of manganese deficiency, a condition in which the body

doesn't have enough manganese. It is also used for weak bones (osteoporosis), a type of "tired blood" (anemia), and symptoms of premenstrual syndrome(PMS).

Manganese is sometimes included with chondroitin sulfate and glucosamine hydrochloride in multi-ingredient products promoted for osteoarthritis. Certain supplements, including those commonly used for osteoarthritis contain manganese.

Warning

When using these products, it's important to follow label directions carefully. At doses slightly higher than the recommended dose, these products provide more than the ***Tolerable Upper Limit*** (UL) for adults, ***11 mg of manganese per day***. Consuming more than 11 mg per day of manganese could cause serious and harmful side effects.

How does it work?

Manganese is an essential nutrient involved in many chemical processes in the body, including processing of cholesterol, carbohydrates, and protein. It might also be involved in bone formation.

WebMD.com

Magnesium

Magnesium is a mineral that is present in relatively large amounts in the body. Researchers estimate that the average person's body contains about 25 grams of magnesium, and about half of that is in the bones. Magnesium is important in more than 300 chemical reactions that keep the body working properly. People get magnesium from their diet, but sometimes magnesium supplements are needed if magnesium levels are too low. Dietary intake of magnesium may be low, particularly among women.

An easy way to remember foods that are good magnesium sources is to think fiber. Foods that are high in fiber are generally high in magnesium. Dietary sources of magnesium include legumes, whole grains, vegetables (especially broccoli, squash, and green leafy vegetables), seeds, and nuts (especially almonds). Other sources include dairy products, meats, chocolate, and coffee. Water with a high mineral content, or "hard" water, is also a source of magnesium.

People take magnesium to prevent or treat magnesium deficiency. Magnesium deficiency is not uncommon in the US. It's particularly common among African Americans and the elderly.

Magnesium is also used as a laxative for constipation and for preparation of the bowel for surgical or diagnostic procedures. It is also used as an antacid for acid indigestion.

Some people use magnesium for diseases of the heart and blood vessels including chest pain, irregular heartbeat, high blood pressure, high levels of "bad" cholesterol called low-density lipoprotein (LDL) cholesterol, low levels of "good" cholesterol called high-density lipoprotein (HDL) cholesterol, heart valve disease (mitral valve prolapse), and heart attack.

Magnesium is also used for treating attention deficit-hyperactivity disorder (ADHD),anxiety, chronic fatigue syndrome (CFS), Lyme disease, fibromyalgia, leg cramps during pregnancy, diabetes, kidney stones, migraine headaches, weak bones (osteoporosis), premenstrual syndrome (PMS), altitude sickness, urinary incontinence, restless leg syndrome, asthma, hay fever, multiple sclerosis, and for preventing hearing loss.

Athletes sometimes use magnesium to increase energy and endurance.

Some people put magnesium on their skin to treat

infected skin ulcers, boils, and carbuncles; and to speed up wound healing. Magnesium is also used as a cold compress in the treatment of a severe skin infection caused by strep bacteria (erysipelas) and as a hot compress for deep-seated skin infections.

Some companies that manufacture magnesium/calcium combination supplements promote a 2:1 or 3:1 ratio as being ideal for absorption of these elements. However, there is no credible research to support this claim. Claims that coral calcium products have ideal combinations of magnesium and calcium to cure a variety of diseases and conditions are being carefully evaluated by the US Food and Drug Administration (FDA) and US Federal Trade Commission (FTC).

How does it work?

Magnesium is required for the proper growth and maintenance of bones. Magnesium is also required for the proper function of nerves, muscles, and many other parts of the body. In the stomach, magnesium helps neutralize stomach acid and moves stools through the intestine.

WebMD.com

Sodium

Sodium, or salt, is a mineral found in many foods, sometimes in very high amounts. The typical American eats much more salt than the body needs. If you're eating more than a pinch of salt a day -- about a teaspoon -- you are eating more than recommended. Too much salt in your diet affects your body's fluid balance and can lead to serious health problems, including high blood pressure and kidney disease. A healthy diet is one that is low in sodium. For most adults that means no more than 1,500 milligrams per day.

WebMD.com

Potassium

Potassium is a mineral that's crucial for life. Potassium is necessary for the heart, kidneys, and other organs to work normally.

Why do people take potassium?

Most people who eat a healthy diet should get enough potassium naturally. However, many Americans don't eat a healthy diet and may be deficient in potassium. Low potassium is associated with a risk of high blood pressure, heart disease, stroke, arthritis, cancer, digestive disorders, and infertility. For people with low potassium, doctors sometimes recommend improved diets -- or potassium supplements -- to prevent or treat some of these conditions.

Potassium deficiencies are more common in people who:

- Use certain medicines, such as diuretics and certain birth control pills
- Have physically demanding jobs
- Are athletes
- Have health conditions that affect their digestive absorption, such as Crohn's disease
- Have an eating disorder
- Smoke
- Abuse alcohol or drugs

How much potassium should you take?

The Institute of Medicine has set an adequate intake for potassium. Getting this amount of potassium from diet, with or without supplements, should be enough to keep you healthy. The FDA has determined that foods that contain at least 350 milligrams of potassium can bear the following label: "Diets containing foods that are good sources of potassium and low in sodium may reduce the risk of high blood pressure and stroke."

Category	Adequate Intake (AI)
CHILDREN	
0-6 months	400 mg/day
7-12 months	700 mg/day
1-3 years	3,000 mg/day
4-8 years	3,800 mg/day
9-13 years	4,500 mg/day
14 years and up	4,700 mg/day
ADULTS	
18 years and up	4,700 mg/day
Pregnant women	4,700 mg/day
Breastfeeding women	5,100 mg/day

Always take potassium supplements with a full glass of water or juice.

There is no set upper limit for potassium. So it's not clear exactly how much potassium you can take safely. However, very high doses of potassium can be deadly.

Can you get potassium naturally from foods?

Good natural food sources of potassium include:

- Bananas
- Avocados
- Nuts, like almonds and peanuts
- Citrus fruits
- Leafy, green vegetables
- Milk
- Potatoes

Keep in mind that some types of cooking, such as boiling, can destroy the potassium in some foods.

What are the risks of taking potassium?

- **Side effects.** At normal doses, potassium is fairly safe. It may cause an upset stomach. Some people have allergies to potassium supplements.

- **Interactions.** Potassium supplements may not be safe if you take certain medicines for diabetes, high blood pressure or heart disease. Check with your doctor first if you take any medications before you take potassium supplements.

- **Warnings.** People with kidney disease, diabetes, heart disease, Addison's disease, stomach ulcers, or other health problems should never take potassium supplements without talking to a doctor first.

- **Overdose.** Signs of a potassium overdose include confusion, tingling sensation in the limbs, low blood pressure, irregular heartbeat, weakness, and coma. Get emergency medical help immediately.

Webmd.com

Selenium

Selenium is a mineral found in the soil. Selenium naturally appears in water and some foods. While people only need a very small amount, selenium plays a key role in the metabolism.

Why do people take selenium?

Selenium has attracted attention because of its antioxidant properties. Antioxidants protect cells from damage. There is some evidence that selenium supplements may reduce the odds of prostate cancer. Selenium does not seem to affect the risk of colorectal or lung cancer. But beware: selenium also seems to *increase* the risk of non-melanoma skin cancer.

Among healthy people in the U.S., selenium deficiencies are uncommon. But some health conditions -- such as HIV, Crohn's disease, and others -- are associated with low selenium levels. People who are fed intravenously are also at risk for low selenium. Doctors sometimes suggest that people with these conditions use selenium supplements.

Selenium has also been studied for the treatment of dozens of conditions. They range from asthma to arthritis to dandruff to infertility. However, the results have been inconclusive.

Group	Recommended Dietary Allowance
Children 1-3	20 micrograms/day
Children 4-8	30 micrograms/day
Children 9-13	40 micrograms/day
Adults and children 14 and up	55 micrograms/day
Pregnant women	60 micrograms/day

Breastfeeding women	70 micrograms/day

How much selenium should you take?

The recommended dietary allowance (RDA) includes the total amount of selenium you should get from foods and from any supplements you take. Most people can get their RDA of selenium from food.

In studies supporting the use of selenium for prostate cancer prevention, men took 200 micrograms daily.

The safe upper limit for selenium is 400 micrograms a day in adults. Anything above that is considered an overdose.

Can you get selenium naturally from foods?

Selenium content of food is largely dependent on location and soil conditions, which vary widely. The average daily intake in the U.S. is 125 mcg per day. Populations of the Eastern Coastal Plain and the Pacific Northwest have the lowest selenium levels, averaging between 60 to 90 mcg per day, which is still considered to be adequate intake.

Good natural food sources of selenium include:

- Nuts, like Brazil nuts and walnuts
- Many fresh and saltwater fish, like tuna, cod, red snapper, and herring
- Beef and poultry
- Grains

Whole foods are the best sources of selenium. The mineral may be destroyed during processing.

What are the risks of taking selenium?

- **Side effects.** Taken at normal doses, selenium does not usually have side effects. An overdose of selenium may cause bad breath, fever, nausea, and liver, kidney and heart problems. At high enough levels, selenium could cause death.

- **Interactions.** Selenium may also interact with other medicines and supplements, such as antacids, chemotherapy drugs, corticosteroids, niacin, cholesterol-lowering statin drugs, and birth control pills.

- **Skin cancer.** Selenium supplements are associated with a risk of skin cancer (squamous cell carcinoma), so people at high risk of skin cancer should not take these supplements.

- **Diabetes.** One study found that people who took 200 micrograms a day of selenium were 50% more likely to develop type 2 diabetes. So far, it's unknown if the selenium actually caused the disease. Discuss the risk with your doctor.

Webmd.com

Herbs

Guarana

Guarana is a plant named for the Guarani tribe in the Amazon, who used the seeds to brew a drink. Today, guarana seeds are still used as medicine.

Guarana is used for weight loss, to enhance athletic performance, as a stimulant, and to reduce mental and physical fatigue. It is a frequent addition to energy and weight loss products.

Some people also use guarana to treat low blood pressure and chronic fatigue syndrome (CFS), and to prevent malaria and dysentery. It is also used to enhance sexual desire, to increase urine flow, and as an astringent.

Other uses include treatment of ongoing diarrhea, fever, heart problems, headache, joint pain, backache, and heat stress.

In food manufacturing, guarana has been used as a flavoring ingredient in beverages and candy.

How does it work?

Guarana contains caffeine. Caffeine works by stimulating the central nervous system (CNS), heart, and muscles. Guarana also contains theophylline and theobromine, which are chemicals similar to caffeine.

Silymarin

Milk thistle is a plant that contains silymarin, a substance that improves liver function. Originally from Europe, milk thistle now also grows in the United States.

You can take milk thistle in capsules or as a tincture (combined with alcohol). It has been widely used in Europe and Germany, where it is a common complementary treatment for liver problems such as hepatitis and cirrhosis. In the United States, it is sold as a dietary supplement.

What is milk thistle used for?

People use milk thistle as a complementary treatment for liver problems, particularly hepatitis and cirrhosis and inflammation of the bile ducts (cholangitis). Research on silymarin suggests that it may protect the liver from inflammation. But it does not have a direct effect on viruses that cause hepatitis, such as the hepatitis C virus.1

Preliminary research suggests that silymarin is an antioxidant, which helps protect the body from cell-destroying substances called free radicals. Silymarin also may reduce inflammation and block the effects of toxins that harm the liver.2

Two studies on milk thistle presented conflicting results. One study found that milk thistle appeared to help some people with cirrhosis live longer than they would have otherwise, while another found no benefit.2

Big review
Food Sources for Vitamins and Minerals

When it comes to vitamins and minerals, you're probably looking for the bottom line: how much do you need? Here's a chart to help you out. It gives you a rundown of all the vitamins and minerals you should get -- preferably from food -- along with details on a couple of other important nutrients and electrolytes.

Note that the recommended amounts of these vitamins and minerals are listed in three different ways: grams, milligrams, and micrograms.

Vitamin or Mineral	Examples of Good Food Sources	What It Does	Recommended Daily Amount (RDA) or Adequate	Upper Limit (The Highest Amount You Can Take Without Risk
Calcium	Milk, yogurt, hard cheeses, fortified cereals, spinach	Essential for bone growth and strength, blood clotting, muscle contraction, and the transmission of nerve signals	**Adults age 19-50:** 1,000 milligrams/day **Adults age 51 and up:** 1,200 milligrams/day	2,500 milligrams/day
Choline (Vitamin B complex)	Milk, liver, eggs, peanuts	Plays a key role in the production of cells and neuro-transmitters	**Men:** 550 milligrams/day **Women:** 425 milligrams/day	3,500 milligrams/day

			Pregnant women: 450 milligrams/day	
			Breastfeeding women: 550 milligrams/day	
Chromium	Meats, poultry, fish, some cereals	Helps control blood sugar levels	**Adult men age 19-50:** 35 micrograms/day **Adult men age 51 and up:** 30 micrograms/day **Adult women age 19-50:** 25 micrograms/day **Adult women age 51 and up:** 20 micrograms/day **Pregnant women:** 30 micrograms/day **Breastfeeding women:** 45 micrograms/day	Unknown

Copper	Seafood, nuts, seeds, wheat bran cereals, whole grains	Important in the metabolism of iron	**Adults:** 900 micrograms/day **Pregnant women:** 1,000 micrograms/day **Breastfeeding women:** 1,300 micrograms/day	10,000 micrograms/ day
Fiber	Bran cereal, peas, lentils, black beans, fruits, vegetables	Helps with digestion and the maintenance of blood sugar levels; reduces the risk of heart disease	**Adult men age 19-50:** 38 grams/day **Adult men age 51 and up:** 30 grams/day **Adult women age 19-50:** 25 grams/day **Adult women age 51 and up:**21 grams/day **Pregnant women:** 28 grams/day **Breastfeeding women:** 29 grams/day	None
Fluoride	Fluoridated water, some sea fish, some toothpastes	Prevents the formation of tooth cavities and stimulates	**Adult men:** 4 milligrams/day **Adult women (including pregnant and**	10 milligrams/day

	and mouth rinses	the growth of bone	**breastfeeding):** 3 milligrams/day	
Folic Acid (Folate)	Dark, leafy vegetables; enriched and whole grain breads; fortified cereals	Key for the development of cells, protein metabolism and heart health; in pregnant women, helps prevent birth defects	**Adults:** 400 micrograms/day **Pregnant women:** 600 micrograms/day **Breastfeeding women:** 500 micrograms/day	1,000 micrograms/ day
Iodine	Processed foods and iodized salt	Important in the production of thyroid hormones	Adults: 150 micrograms/day Pregnant women: 220 micrograms/day Breastfeeding women: 290 micrograms/day	1,100 micrograms/ day
Iron	Fortified cereals, beans, lentils, beef, eggs	Key component of red blood cells and many enzymes	**Men:** 8 mg/day **Women age 19-50:** 18 mg/day **Women age 51 and up:** 8 mg/day **Pregnant**	45 milligrams/da

			women: 27 mg/day **Breastfeeding women**: 9 mg/day	
Magnesium	Green leafy vegetables, Brazil nuts, almonds, soybeans, halibut, quinoa	Helps with heart rhythm, muscle and nerve function, bone strength	**Adult men age 19-30:** 400 milligrams/day **Adult men age 31 and up:** 420 mg/day **Adult women age 19-30:** 310 milligrams/day Adult women age 31 and up: 320 mg/day **Pregnant women:** 350-360 mg/day **Breastfeeding women:** 310-320 mg/day	For magnesium in food and water, there is no upper limit. For magnesium in supplements or fortified foods 350 milligrams/day
Manganese	Nuts, beans and other legumes, tea, whole grains	Important in forming bones and some enzymes	**Men:** 2.3 mg/day **Adult women:** 1.8 mg/day **Pregnant women:** 2.0 milligrams/day **Breastfeeding**	11 milligrams/day

			women: 2.6 milligrams/day	
Molybden um	Legumes, grains, nuts	Key in the production of some enzymes	**Adults:** 45 micrograms/day **Pregnant and breastfeeding women:** 50 micrograms/day	2,000 micrograms/ day
Phosphoru s	Milk and other dairy products, peas, meat, eggs, some cereals and breads	Allows cells to function normally; helps the body produce energy; key in bone growth	**Adults:** 700 milligrams/day	**Adults up to age 70:** 4,000 milligrams/da **Adults over age 70:** 3,000 milligrams/da **Pregnant women:** 3500 milligrams/da **Breastfeedin women:** 4,000 milligrams/da
Potassium	Sweet potato, bananas, yogurt, yellowfin tuna, soybeans	Important in maintaining normal fluid balance; helps control blood pressure; reduces risk of kidney stones	**Adults:** 4,700 milligrams per day **Breastfeeding women:** 5,100 milligrams/day	Unknown

Selenium	Organ meats, seafood, some plants (if grown in soil with selenium) Brazil nuts.	Protects cells from damage; regulates thyroid hormone	**Adults:** 55 micrograms/day **Pregnant women:** 60 micrograms/day **Breastfeeding women:** 70 micrograms/day	400 micrograms/day
Sodium	Foods to which sodium chloride (salt) has been added, like salted meats, nuts, butter, and a vast number of processed foods	Important for fluid balance	**Adults age 19-50:** 1500 milligrams/day **Adults age 51-70:** 1,300 milligrams/day **Adults age 71 and up:** 1,200 milligrams/day	2,300 milligrams/day
Vitamin A	Sweet potato with peel, carrots, spinach, fortified cereals	Necessary for normal vision, immune function, reproduction	**Men:** 900 micrograms/day **Women:** 700 micrograms/day	3,000 micrograms/day

Vitamin B$_1$(Thiamin)	Whole grain, enriched, fortified products; bread; cereals	Allows the body to process carbohydrates and some protein.	**Men: 1.2** milligrams/day **Women: 1.1** milligrams/day **Pregnant and breastfeeding women: 1.4** milligrams/day	Unknown
Vitamin B$_2$(Riboflavin)	Milk, bread products, fortified cereals	Key in metabolism and the conversion of food into energy; helps produce red blood cells	Men: 1.3 milligrams/day Women: 1.1 milligrams/day Pregnant Women: 1.4 milligrams/day Breastfeeding Women: 1.6 milligrams/day	Unknown
Vitamin B$_3$(Niacin)	Meat, fish, poultry, enriched and whole grain breads, fortified cereals	Assists in digestion and the conversion of food into energy; important in the production of cholesterol	**Men: 16** milligrams/day **Women: 14** milligrams/day **Pregnant Women: 18** milligrams/day **Breastfeeding women: 17** milligrams/day	For niacin in natural source there is no upper limit. For niacin in supplements o fortified foods 35 milligrams/da

Vitamin B$_5$ (Pantothenic Acid)	Chicken, beef, potatoes, oats, cereals, tomatoes	Important in fatty acid metabolism	**Adults:** 5 milligrams/day **Pregnant women:** 6 milligrams/day **Breastfeeding women:** 7 milligrams/day	Unknown
Vitamin B$_6$	Fortified cereals, fortified soy products, organ meats	Important for the nervous system; helps the body metabolize proteins and sugar	**Men age 19-50:** 1.3 milligrams/day **Men age 51 up:** 1.7 milligrams/day **Women age 19-50:** 1.3 milligrams/day **Women age 51 up:** 1.5 milligrams/day **Pregnant women:** 1.9 milligrams/day **Breastfeeding women:** 2 milligrams/day	100 milligrams/day
Vitamin B$_7$ (Biotin)	Liver, fruits, meats	Helps with the synthesis of fats, glycogen and amino acids	**Adults:** 30 micrograms/day **Breastfeeding women:** 35 micrograms/day	Unknown

Vitamin B$_{12}$(Cobalamin)	Fish, poultry, meat, fortified cereals	Important in the production of red blood cells	**Adults:** 2.4 micrograms/day **Pregnant women:** 2.6 micrograms/day **Breastfeeding women:** 2.8 micrograms/day	Unknown
Vitamin C	Red and green peppers, kiwis, oranges, strawberries, broccoli	Antioxidant that protects against cell damage, boosts the immune system, forms collagen in the body	**Men:** 90 milligrams/day **Women:** 75 milligrams/day **Pregnant women:** 85 milligrams/day **Breastfeeding women:** 120 milligrams/day	2,000 milligrams/day
Vitamin D (Calciferol)	Fish liver oils, fatty fish, fortified milk products, fortified cereals; also, formed naturally as a result of sunlight exposure	Crucial in metabolizing calcium for healthy bones	**Adults age 18-50:** 5 micrograms/day **Adults age 51-70:** 10 micrograms/day **Adults over age 70:** 15 micrograms/day **Pregnant and breastfeeding women:** 5 micrograms/day	50 microgram day

Vitamin E (alpha-tocopherol)	Fortified cereals, sunflower seeds, almonds, peanut butter, vegetable oils	Antioxidant that protects cells against damage	**Adults (including pregnant women):** 15 milligrams/day **Breastfeeding women:** 19	1,000 milligrams/day
Vitamin K	Green vegetables like spinach, collards, and broccoli; brussels sprouts; cabbage	Important in blood clotting and bone health	**Men:** 120 micrograms/day —— **Women (including pregnant and breastfeeding):** 90 micrograms/day	Unknown
Zinc	Red meats, some seafood, fortified cereals	Supports the body's immunity and nerve function; important in reproduction	**Men:** 11 milligrams/day —— **Women:** 8 milligrams/day **Pregnant women:** 11 milligrams/day **Breastfeeding**	40 milligrams/day

			women: 12 milligrams/day	

Final Thoughts

I became convinced after reading Outliers by Malcolm Gladwell that the secret to longevity is balance. There is not one single gene, or food item, or ritual which increases likelihood of longevity like balance.

Manage stress. Stress is stuff out of our control. Control your body and do some exercise. Negative effects of stress are reduced.

It is not important how many days you accumulate in this present form. With good health, though, there will be many benefits.

Notes, Things to Buy, Etc.

_____

_____

_____

_____

_____

_____

_____

_____

_____

_____

_____

Index

(Fill in the blanks with topics of interest and
corresponding page number)

Questions and Comments for Author

To help make this a better book in future editions please email ideas to vincentrdegruy@msn.com

Mention the book in the subject line.